Care Aesthetics

What if the work of a nurse, physio, or homecare worker was designated an art, so that the qualities of the experiences they create became understood as aesthetic qualities? What if the interactions and physical connections created by artists, directors, dancers, or workshop facilitators was understood as a work of care? *Care Aesthetics* is the first full-length book to explore these questions and examine the work of carer artists and artist carers to make the case for the importance of valuing and supporting aesthetically caring relations across multiple aspects of our lives.

Theoretically and practically, the book outlines the implications of care aesthetics for the socially engaged arts field and health and social care, and for acts of aesthetic care in the everyday. Part 1 of the book outlines the approaches to aesthetics and to care theory that are necessary to make and defend the concept of care aesthetics. Part 2 then tests this through practice, examining socially engaged arts and health and social care through its lens. It makes the case for careful art exploring the implications of care aesthetics for participatory or applied arts. Then it argues for artful care and how an aesthetic orientation to care practices might challenge some of the inadequacies of contemporary care.

This is a vital, paradigm-shifting book for anyone engaged with socially engaged arts or social and health care practices on an academic or professional level.

James Thompson is Professor of Applied Theatre at the University of Manchester, where he has held senior roles, most recently as Vice President for Social Responsibility. He was the co-founder of the Theatre in Prisons and Probation Centre, the arts organisation, *In Place of War*, and has run arts projects in conflict zones internationally. He has written widely on applied theatre and the socially engaged arts.

Care Aesthetics

For artful care and careful art

James Thompson

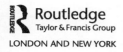
Routledge
Taylor & Francis Group

LONDON AND NEW YORK

Cover image: Pekic/Getty Image

First published 2023
by Routledge
4 Park Square, Milton Park, Abingdon, Oxon OX14 4RN

and by Routledge
605 Third Avenue, New York, NY 10158

Routledge is an imprint of the Taylor & Francis Group, an informa business

© 2023 James Thompson

British Library Cataloguing-in-Publication Data
A catalogue record for this book is available from the British Library

Library of Congress Cataloging-in-Publication Data
A catalog record has been requested for this book

ISBN: 9781032196176 (hbk)
ISBN: 9781032196169 (pbk)
ISBN: 9781003260066 (ebk)

DOI: 10.4324/9781003260066

Typeset in Bembo
by KnowledgeWorks Global Ltd.

To Mum, Frances, with love

Contents

Acknowledgements

All writing is indebted to a dialogue with others and this book is no exception. For Care Aesthetics, I want to thank family, friends, and colleagues for inspiring and directly contributing to the process of the book's development. This includes my friends and partners in the Democratic Republic of the Congo who perhaps unbeknownst to them shifted my thinking and prepared the early ground for this work. In particular, the much-missed Eraste Rwatangabo and Antoine Muvunyi who still lives and works in Uvira, South Kivu. Many people read early drafts and provided invaluable criticism. Maggie Gale, a colleague close to home at the University of Manchester, was generous with her time and ever helpful in her detailed feedback on the work. Cindy Cohen, at Brandeis University, Massachusetts, a little further away, has been hugely supportive – her insightful comments on one of the early chapters was vital for its development. Maggie and Cindy are exemplary colleagues, and I cannot thank them enough for their friendship and good-humoured conversations over many years. Similarly, I want to thank Paul Heritage, from Queen Mary, University of London and People's Palace Projects who provided invaluable guidance on an early draft. It goes without saying that the many colleagues at Taylor and Francis have made the process of getting this work from idea to print so much easier. I want to thank Ben Piggot for his commitment to the project and Steph Hines for her professional support throughout the process.

Much of this book was completed during the pandemic while I was on sabbatical from my university. I want to thank the many colleagues at Manchester who made this possible, in particular all colleagues from the Drama Department and notably the current head of department, Jenny Hughes. She demonstrated amazing leadership at this difficult time and made the struggles that many faced during the multiple lockdowns that much easier to manage. While away on sabbatical, I had the privilege of working in Portugal and I would like to thank the many colleagues there for their kindness and hospitality. Isabel Bezelga at the University of Évora, Hugo Cruz co-founder of the Associação MEXE from Porto, António Vicente from Teatro Imediato, O Grupo de Teatro Terapêutico do Hospital Júlio de Matos and Teatro de Identidades in Lisbon, and Isabel Menezes from the University of Porto. While working in Portugal, I had the fortune to stay with Bev and Etienne Wenger-Traynor and want to thank them for their welcome and their willingness to open their house to me. Writing from their home was a constant joy and provided a great space to focus on the process of reworking the book.

I want to thank people I engaged with during the writing who inspired it in different ways. Amanda Stuart Fisher, from the Royal Central School of Speech and Drama, has been a co-conspirator on all things related to performance and care. She was the co-editor of our book *Performing Care* which was a rehearsal for several the ideas in this book, and I want to acknowledge that some of the words here have been borrowed from that edition. Maurice Hamington, from Portland State University, has been a great support and his work on *embodied care* frames much of my approach to care ethics as explained in Chapter 2. I want to thank Roger Robinson and Peepal Tree Press for their permission to quote his poem 'Grace' from his collection *A Portable Paradise* (2019), which is central to the introduction to the book. Clive Parkinson who is a great artist and thinker in the field of arts and health and always offers wise words for anyone seeking to bring together work in health, care, and the arts. Peter Jenkinson and Shelagh Wright are great friends and two of the best arts and social provocateurs who have provided me with endless links and contacts that have been vital for many of the debates in these pages. In a different way, Dawn Cheshire and her son Connor have been friends throughout the pandemic and I want to acknowledge how much her bright and curious lad taught me about care (and cake!). Then Jenny Harris and Ric Demby – great friends and enduring source of support. They provided vital and generous discussion about the arts, care, and the political woes facing our country, particularly during the endless weeks of lockdown.

Care Aesthetics is the subject of a research project funded by the UK Arts and Humanities Research Council, and I want to thank them for the support for the project. The research team behind this project have been important inspiration behind the ideas in this book and I am excited about the work we are developing together. Thanks to John Keady, Professor of Mental Health Nursing at University of Manchester; Jackie Kindell, Visiting Lecturer at Manchester and Head of Allied Health Professionals and Social Workers at Pennine Care NHS Foundation Trust; and Kerry Harman, Senior Lecturer in the Department of Psychosocial Studies at Birkbeck, University of London.

Finally, I want to thank my family – Mum Francis, sister Bridget and partner Kevin in Goring, nieces Molly in Barcelona, Evie in Manchester and Danya in Newcastle, parents-in-law Stan and Judy in Ilkley, and then sister-in-law and brother-in-law Sharon and Paul in Leeds. Love and thanks always to daughters Hannah and Leah, in London and Manchester, respectively, and my wife, partner, and love of my life, Debbie, here in Chorlton. Conversations (URL and IRL) and care from all of you have been indispensable across the time it has taken to write this book. A last thanks to my future grandchild, who as I type this has been making my daughter Hannah feel lousy – I know you will be a focus for future care from all those who already love you.

Excerpt from 'Grace', *A Portable Paradise* (Peepal Tree Press, 2019) © Roger Robinson, reproduced by permission of Peepal Tree Press.

Introduction

Care aesthetics is an idea that makes a double claim. First, it speaks to my home field of applied theatre or socially engaged arts. It argues that we need to think how the making of art can be an act of care. Care is not a context, a theme or a set of protocols governing practice. Instead, the book argues that through the process of working with people, materials, and places, care happens: as a game is played or as we rehearse and stage a performance, care takes place. The second claim flips this first one. It says that caring, whether in formal health and social care settings, or informally in the activity that many of us are involved in our daily lives, can be an aesthetic practice: that is, it has a certain craft and involves the creation of sensory, embodied experiences. This book is an investigation of these related claims. Care aesthetics applies equally to arts practices and care processes – to the work of a theatre facilitator and a health care assistant – and there is, therefore, a deliberate attempt to blur professional and practice-based boundaries. The implications of this will be discussed in the pages that follow.

I start with three short accounts. They are used to introduce the approach to the chapters that follow. They discuss in turn a personal anecdote, a poem, and a chapter from a book.

The anecdote

When my colleague from the Democratic Republic of the Congo, Antoine Muvunyi, came to the UK, and was still learning English, he turned to me one day and said, 'James, why in England do people put their children in wheelbarrows?' He could not understand why parents pushed their children onto buses or trams and then had them facing away from them, nestled in the *wheelbarrow*, while they busied themselves looking at their phones. Antoine Muvunyi will be a character who appears a number of times in the pages that

DOI: 10.4324/9781003260066-1

follow, and in fact was introduced in my first writing on 'an aesthetics of care' (Thompson, 2015). He was a friend and collaborator from the Congo, who was shot while working on a theatre and women's rights project, and he spent over six months living with me and my family during his recuperation. His treatment and care will be mentioned in more detail later, but this insight from Antoine provides a starting point to illustrate perspectives on care that run through this edition.

My proper response to *why do you put your children in wheelbarrows*, was not 'those are pushchairs, buggies, strollers, not wheelbarrows' because his choice of words was actually wonderfully telling about a norm of care that deserved to be questioned. He did not ask this question with a sense of superiority but of genuine concern for both the child, but more particularly for the relations we were developing with our offspring. Of course, this is not to reify the child rearing practices in Antoine's home country, but to note that asking questions about the way we care reveals dynamics that are often unnoticed. Care is not a fixed, unchanging, or culturally static practice, but shifts in response to different contexts, cultures, and times. Care changes in the eye of the beholder and any analysis of care must acknowledge that it is always embedded in certain cultural norms and expectations. This book does not present a case for *good* care but argues that there are many forms of good and bad care, that are often hard to perceive from within certain contexts. Antoine revealed the importance of seeing care from different cultural perspectives but also his gentle admonishment illustrated that commenting on the practices of care can also be a socio-cultural critique. We do put our children in wheelbarrows that face away from their parents, and we need to reflect on what this both says about our society but also more importantly for this book, what it creates: what relations are produced and reproduced in this process. In noting the form and responding with a sense of genuine anxiety to our tendency to use wheelbarrows in this way, Antoine was also making a comment on the aesthetics of the care we take of our children. So, a focus on aesthetics teaches us about micro relations that are important for the quality of our lives but also points to how attention to the quality of care is a powerful means for critiquing the way our human-to-human relations are practiced and produced.

This book will use anecdotes – stories from my and other people's personal and professional experience that raise issues about care. These insist that our practice and our interpretation of care is always partial and situated in specific local, culturally particular, and historically unique contexts. They are also used to emphasise that care is not something over there, done by others and separate from our lives. Giving and receiving care is part and parcel of all our lives and therefore my own involvement in care will, at times, feature in the pages that follow. If in the text, I claim that the care was *beautiful* or *ugly*, I fully accept that this is a partial interpretation dependent on the particular context from which I live and work. I might be describing pushchairs; others might see wheelbarrows.

The poem

Roger Robinson is a poet and performer who lives and works between London in the UK and Trinidad in the Caribbean. His poetry collection *A Portable Paradise* (2019) won the 2020 T.S. Eliot prize and offers a remarkable journey through different visions of utopia in contemporary British life. It is both affirming about the endurance of a Black-British experience, a blast against the inequities of events like the Grenfell Tower disaster and a moving account of moments of care. His poem *Grace* in the collection has been called by him in public readings a *love story to the NHS and its nurses* and it tells the story of the care for his premature son by a particular Jamaican nurse. I happily admit it is my favourite poem in the collection and here I quote the final two stanzas:

> Another consultant tells the nurses to stop feeding a baby,
> who will soon die,
> and she commands her loyal nurses to feed him. "No baby must dead
> wid a hungry belly." And she'd sit in the dark, rocking that
> well-fed baby,
> held to her bosom, slowly humming the melody of "Happy" by Pharrell.
> And I think, if by some chance, I'm not here and my son's life
> should flicker,
> then Grace, she should be the one. (2019: 69)

Care Aesthetics will use many examples from the arts, and because of my background these will mostly be from the area of socially engaged or participatory theatre. As I said above, the relation I am discussing is not art *about* care or art *in* care settings but the art *of* care – and why I choose to use the word *aesthetics* is explained in detail in Chapter 1. That said, *Grace* is a poem *about* care. The reason this particular artwork is an important starting point for the book however is that Robinson illustrates a number of the central concerns of care aesthetics. First, Grace holds, rocks and sings. The poem is quietly noting and celebrating the aesthetics of her caring practice. She demonstrates an attention to her charge, a precision of movement and bodily action, and shows her profound understanding of the intimate relation between music and comfort. As will be discussed in subsequent chapters, these are elements of care aesthetics in practice. She does not add bodily movement and music on top of her care for the infant, they are integrated parts of it.

There are two other reasons for introducing this poem. One is that this type of care is done *in spite of* a demand to the contrary. Grace refuses the instruction of the consultant and commands her nurses to do exactly the opposite. When this edition points at 'good' care, or beautifully crafted caring responses, it seeks to validate it as a practice that is often resistant. Quality care can compete with norms that push in an opposite direction. The book is not simply an account of care aesthetics as a 'nice to have', it is the case for care aesthetics as an important part of caring that responds to contexts where care is too often poor.

Care aesthetics is evaluative as well as descriptive, and in its evaluative form it is meant to be a critique of the inadequacies and cruelties that exist in many careless contexts.

My final point is that Robinson describes Grace as a 'Jamaican senior nurse', and it is important to note that care can never be detached from specifics of the life experiences of its practitioners. We cannot separate the caring practices of the UK's National Health Service from the patterns of migration that have forged it and the cultures of care that many different communities brought to it. Care is shaped at a minimum by differences in race, gender and class and in focusing on the aesthetics of care it seeks to value the subtle differences in capacity and skill brought by diverse communities. This is not to say that care aesthetics is a practice that belongs to a certain community or is in any way 'natural' to any particular group. It is an argument that care is often a set of practices that are undervalued because of failures to recognise those people who undertake care and support others. Care Aesthetics, the book, is about shining a firm light on those practices of exceptional virtuosity so often overlooked in many contemporary accounts of 'professional' care and 'professional' arts. It asserts the significance and importance of the astounding aesthetic experience created by carers who are often poorly paid, rarely acknowledged and too often side-lined by hierarchies of value linked to types of formal and informal labour. If this book needs an exemplar of what it is trying to capture and champion, how care will feed babies in spite of the orders of others and do it with a warm hold and song of happiness, *then Grace, she should be the one.*

The book acknowledges the disparities and injustices that are caused by inequalities based on gender, race, class and, as the next example demonstrates, sexuality. Care Aesthetics recognises that care is poorly distributed, rewarded, and valued, but sees poems such as *Grace* as part of a project to bring recognition to the astounding craft by which it is often executed.

The chapter

In 2020, the Boston Review and Verso Books brought out the collection called '*The Politics of Care: From COVID-19 to Black Lives Matter*' edited by Deborah Chasman and Joshua Cohen. It makes the bold argument, summarised on its back cover, that the *greatest social crisis of a generation* which we are currently living through, needs a *new kind of* politics, and that is *a politics of care*. While Care Aesthetics sees itself as part of this political response and is adamant that the focus on aesthetics is part of a political account of the importance of care and not a distraction from it, it is one particular chapter which I will draw attention to here. It is written by activist, writer and former editor of Boston's Gay Community News, Amy Hoffman. I choose this chapter, poignantly titled *Love One Another or Die*, to point to the importance of recognising the different ways that care is both written about and materialises in people's lives. Hoffman's chapter reflects on the history of the Lesbian and Gay communities of Boston, the lives affected by a network of bars, meeting places, private parties, and of course the Stonewall riots and oppressive policing. She was features editor on the Gay Community News in 1979 when they put together the Stonewall tenth anniversary edition. Her writing takes us through stories of public campaigning and personal caring, particularly of friends with HIV/AIDS. She documents the movement as it moved from the 'Lesbian and Gay' community to the broader LGBTQ+ and queer politics of more recent years. What I want to draw attention to here is that when we focus on today's pandemic and discuss the extraordinary impact it has had on many people, we should not forget that for certain communities a pandemic, and a crisis of care, is not a new thing. She writes that living through today's 'terrifying pandemic' has given her time to 'reflect on the early days of queer liberation and that other pandemic' (2020: 51).

That other pandemic reminds us that care crises have histories, they have antecedents, and we should learn from them and acknowledge that pandemics bring with them a long history of discrimination and response to that discrimination. Hoffman's account is important because it shifts between a public and private register, demonstrating that the work of caring for friends and caring for a community wove back and forth between each other. The appalling treatment of patients with HIV/AIDS was a public disgrace but was experienced through the daily practices of intimate care. As Hoffman tells the story of persuading people *not to wear gloves* when meeting people with AIDS, we see love and care as part of the struggle against homophobia and injustice. And importantly, the look and feel of wearing gloves compared to caring for someone without them produces a different sensation, a different aesthetic of that care. The practice of caring intimately for your friends was for Hoffman part of 'what it was like to live as a community under siege' and 'Gay Liberation' for her was marked by 'how we rose to the challenge of caring for one another' (Ibid: 52). Care Aesthetics places itself in a tradition which sees care as connected to broader politics and cannot be relegated to an activity of a disconnected private realm. Who we care for, how we care for them, and what motivates that care, cannot be detached from wider politics that struggles against discrimination and cruelty. The act of care for others and accepting our need to be cared for are part of the way we meet the challenges of different forms of injustice.

The book will use chapters and articles written by a range of commentators, practitioners and academics that shape the way care is debated and documented. The ambition is that these place care and aesthetics in different theoretical and practical traditions and remind us that what we live through today has a long history. There have been many pandemics, and while COVID will appear in these pages, the book acknowledges the words of Amy Hoffman when she urges us to look at others. While it is a huge shift in context, this is echoed by Indigenous leader Takumã Kuikuro of the Kuikuro, from the Xingu indigenous territory of the Amazon region, when in a news report from the early days of the COVID crisis, responded to a question about what he thought of the pandemic by asking 'which one?' Care does not escape its histories, and the terrifying legacies of its absence.

An anecdote, a poem and a chapter. Narrative accounts, artistic practice and academic texts will all inform the pages that follow as I explore how the arts care, and care has a certain artistry. And then, how these two realms relate to each other.

Who the book is for?

The book addresses the socially engaged arts community, applied theatre practitioners, and writers, community-based performance activists and scholars and the huge range of artists who work collaboratively within different groups. This is in many ways my *home* community and I am therefore speaking to colleagues to suggest that care and theories of care are an important lens to consider our practice. Many of us work within care settings, on themes of care, with carers and people who are cared for – and the book values the expertise and experience of many who have developed these practices over decades. The simple assertion here is that it is productive to orientate this work so that making art with people and people making art can be acts of care in themselves.

The book also addresses the care ethics community, drawing on its long history of feminist scholarship and activism, to start from an acceptance of a politics that values interdependence and reciprocity as a source of social good rather than the many contemporary forms of political culture that value strident individualism. Care ethics is the focus of Chapter 2, and the approach here is to accept its premise that an attention to caring relations can be a source of ethics and a means of noting inequalities in caring labour, and how campaigning against injustice does not dismiss care, but seeks to build on the patterns of interhuman care as a source of new forms of sociality and community strength. Care Aesthetics aims to make a contribution to the field of care ethics and takes up the challenge of understanding its sensory and embodied elements. It then seeks to argue that aesthetics can be productively woven into care ethics.

Finally, the book addresses informal and formal carers – health and social care professionals, and in a more extended way those who are cared for and care in their daily lives. It does not aim to bring aesthetics 'to' these practices or fields – it claims that the practice of care already has an aesthetic and focusing on that craft of care, reveals and hopefully champions the extraordinary skills of those who care and the reciprocal responses of those that receive it.

The moment we are in

While the case for care aesthetics has a broad ambition, the discussion in the pages that follow is shaped by the context from which it is written. The book comes from the UK at a time of a pandemic, and therefore it acknowledges the partialities of care and art making here. Most of my examples are relatively local to me, and there is no attempt to suggest they are exemplary. They are the responses within the context of a particular culture and economy of health and social care, a certain history of the socially engaged art and a set of political peculiarities that link to but do not overlap entirely with concerns in other countries. Author and journalist Madeleine Bunting, in her book on the crisis of care in the UK, strikes an optimistic note about this context when she suggests '[w]e could be on the cusp of a dramatic moment when the cultural value of care could be completely recast' (2020: 227). While I am reticent to endorse her optimism entirely, Care Aesthetics accepts the challenge and aims to make a modest contribution to Bunting's *dramatic moment*. Whether the recasting will be in the way we might hope, only time will tell.

Care Aesthetics is an account of the benefit of developing more artful care and careful art, and ultimately an argument for the distinction between them to end. It is shaped by the events of 2020 and 2021, but of course is also part of a history of socially engaged arts practice and scholarship, of the feminist research on the ethics of care, and then long-standing scholarship in the fields of health and social care. It seeks to reaffirm the practice of care as a preeminent location for ethical concerns, but then extends this to argue that it can also be a powerful source of aesthetic experience. The book focuses on the meaning of aesthetics, on how to define care and then how care aesthetics, the concept, might be applied to the socially engaged arts, health and social care and finally everyday life. Care Aesthetics is both an argument for a certain type of aesthetically careful practical experience but also a proposal that we search for and create new examples that might enhance different aspects of our lives.

Before I start that process of *recasting*, however, this introduction will return to some of the arguments in earlier work to give a brief background to the current focus. Much of my previous work has been in the area of theatre and performance studies called 'applied theatre' or 'socially engaged arts', and while this book is connected to these fields, it is also an extension and then departure from them. I started an earlier book, *Performance Affects* (2009), with an account of an evening of singing and dancing during a course I was running in Sri Lanka. I made the straightforward point that where my focus might have traditionally been the theatre workshops exploring issues related to the war in that part of the island, it was the post-workshop cultural practices that hinted at a more inclusive understanding of the role of the arts in this particular context. I extended outwards from the workshops to the more everyday practices of music and dance that I had tended to overlook previously. Care Aesthetics is an attempt to take that shift in a different direction. Rather than the move that suggested the arts in all areas of life are worthy of attention — as *artistic responses to conflict* — here I am making a different move to argue that aesthetic experience happens in the workshops, the evening's entertainment, and also in many other everyday practices that are far more expansive than those that might be contained under the category understood as *the arts*. A focus on aesthetic experiences across multiple life practices does not seek to dismiss the importance of the arts per se but consider them as only one category of practices that offer important aesthetic experiences that contribute to people's lives. Artistic experience may be particularly strong, bold or acutely felt, but it is embedded in life practices many of which have different levels of aesthetic richness or depth. This book explores those aesthetic experiences that take place within moments care, whether human to human, amongst groups of people, between people and objects or their wider world. The extension here is, therefore, from applied theatre to the aesthetic experience of care in multiple life settings: some of which might of course be part of traditional applied theatre programmes, and many of which are not.

Performance Affects asked how we might explore those *affective* aspects of the arts to argue that a *socially engaged practice* must include accounts of the embodied and sensory experiences in art making, and not only those that operate in a register of effect and effectiveness towards some hoped for social outcome. Care Aesthetics develops this emphasis to ask how life sustaining social practices in varied contexts might be understood for the embodied and sensory elements they are composed of and how attention to these aspects of practice might lead to improvements in the quality of interhuman and social relations. This is not attention beyond the aesthetic to a concern with the social, but an argument that the social itself has an aesthetic. So, whether in the context of a participatory art practice or health care in a hospital ward, new opportunities for care-filled life practices become possible through an awareness of the aesthetics of those relations.

If that previous book was written partly in response to my practical work with theatre and performance projects in conflict zones, this book originally intended to explore similar practices in which I was involved. It was planned as an account of examples of projects demonstrating the aesthetics of care, created by artists *and* by health and social care workers in different health and care settings, some of which I would have developed. While it does still offer examples of practice, particularly in part two of the book, these became in the course of the writing somewhat at a distance from my direct experience of them. As mentioned above, this was a result of the context through which the book was written – that of the extended restrictions and multiple lockdowns of the UK's response to the coronavirus pandemic from early 2020 until the middle of 2021. It was a paradoxical process. I was writing of the importance of the aesthetics of caring relations, of the importance of the body and touch in maintaining quality relations between people, in the time of social distancing and enforced isolation. In some ways, this has made the book more cerebral, less practically orientated than I would have hoped. The context of a book's production – for me largely an office in my home in which I worked like many of my compatriots for months with limited journeys outside – shaped what it became. I cannot apologise for the end result, it is what it is, but I do acknowledge the difference in outcome. Of course, the backdrop of a global crisis in care, shaped many of themes as they emerged. Sometimes this is explicit, and at times it is an implicit heightened sense of both the importance of interhuman connection and care, and the terrible results for when it is either absent or poorly distributed. Care Aesthetics is ultimately framed by COVID as a demand for more sensorily rich, well-crafted and nourishing caring relations between people as a counter to the inequalities and injustices of health and care so starkly revealed during the months of lockdown. It forcefully says that artists have a role to play in building and sustaining more care for each other and more care for our world, but crucially extends this to argue that formal and informal carers in multiple contexts can be the inspiration for what a more aesthetically rich form of care giving might look and feel like. All said, in being focused on the importance of care the book too was yearning for more physical examples of care to draw from, and this absence does perhaps hover as a feint loss across the text here.

Above I mention the character of Grace from Roger Robinson's poem and note the aesthetics of the care that she gave the infant in her care. Her singing, her rocking and holding of that child illustrated an aesthetic of care where the boundary between a care practice and an aesthetic experience was properly indistinct. If I am looking for an exemplar of care aesthetics in action *then Grace*, as I say above, *she should be the one*. There are, however, others who will appear in the pages that follow. Another already mentioned is Antoine Muvunyi, who is part of the origin story I bring to care aesthetics and is returned to at a number of points across this work. The story of the care experienced between him and his physiotherapist appears in the opening pages of Chapter 1, and I have written elsewhere (Thompson, 2015) about how this stimulated my first interest in the possibility of reading this relation aesthetically. It was the experience of caring for someone who had undergone a life changing event, that was the grounding for my personal shift from an interest in the role of the arts in conflict zones to one focused on care. It sharpened a realisation that my research and practice had been focused on suffering but too little on what human endeavour might be adequate to meet the challenges of moving beyond it. The American cultural and political theorist, bell hooks, counsels us that 'it is far easier to talk about loss than it is about love' (2001, xxvi) and a shift to *care* is perhaps my response. It is a modest attempt to talk in a different register from one solely grounded in loss. Care Aesthetics is inspired by individuals and relationships where acts of repair do not necessarily solve past injustices or pain, but at least start the processes of creating new networks of embodied relationships that might provide a bulwark against further injury. They might also create joyful collaborations that can sustain stronger connections and mutual support between community members. hooks continues her thesis on love by arguing that 'it is easier to articulate the pain of love's absence than to describe its presence and meaning in our lives' (Ibid). Care Aesthetics responds to her challenge by seeking out a way of starting not from pain, but from describing something of that love, one aspect of which is how more careful and caring experiences can become present and bring meaning to different lives.

Book structure

Part one of the book draws on writing and debate in two areas of scholarship, aesthetics and care, and makes the theoretical case for care aesthetics. The first argument is that human relations can be considered for their aesthetics, and the second is that care is an important source for ethics which can also be understood as an embodied or sensory practice. Chapter 1 focuses on aesthetics and addresses the question as to what is meant by *aesthetics* in the term *care aesthetics*. It considers which aesthetic theories need to be in place, and which in turn need to be rejected for the claim that an apparently social process such as care might be understood as an aesthetic experience. While this chapter is speaking to many within the arts, it aims to be of interest also to those from health and social care, who want to understand why the word 'aesthetics' has been chosen. The second chapter asks the complimentary question as to what is meant by *care* in the term *care aesthetics*. It explores how the history and current debates in the field of care ethics, provide a point of departure for the claim that care can also be understood aesthetically. Again, some of this material might be familiar to care ethicists and those working in the care field, but there is an important extension in making the claim that care can be 'craft-like' or 'artful'. Readers familiar with aesthetic theories might skip sections of Chapter 1 and head to Chapter 2 for more information about care. Those familiar with the care literature might do the reverse. Inevitability when writing across two disciplinary areas, some sections might be too introductory for some readers, but new for others.

Both these chapters offer largely theoretical accounts to ground the case for care aesthetics that will then be drawn on for the rest of the book. It is worth pointing out here that they have a subtle difference in approach. The first, on aesthetics, is writing against the grain of much aesthetic theory, to make its case that human-to-human relations are a legitimate site of aesthetic experience. In many ways it returns to the origins of aesthetic theory, where aesthetics is a study of sensory perception, before it becomes an approach to the arts. This is of course not new to many in the socially engaged arts and many of the accounts of aesthetics that are both explicit and implicit in debates in this literature are endorsed. The second chapter, on the other hand, writes with the grain of much care ethics theory, accepting it as a productive orientation to how individuals, communities and societies might determine the contours of the ethical relations between them. It is, therefore, written in support of many of the assumptions of feminist care ethicists, rather than arguing with them. It does, of course, take a perspective on this fast-developing field, in particular in the way it pays attention to those care ethicists who work on the theme of embodiment. It uses a turn to embodiment as a link to my case that care ethics also needs to recognise that the sensory actions of the body have an important connection to aesthetics.

Part two of the book examines the concept care aesthetics in practice. Chapter 3, Careful Art, presents the case for the importance of care for the field of socially engaged arts, particularly those involving participatory processes. It offers examples of practice that illustrate care aesthetics, including community dance, one-to-one performance and the playing of theatre games. It then seeks to demonstrate how a focus on care aesthetics questions some of the orientations in socially engaged arts practice, and how attention to an aesthetics of care in the design and delivery of projects is not a retreat from properly risk-taking practice, but a necessary counter to the dislocations and disruptions already faced by many in our contemporary over-individualistic world. The chapter is descriptive in that it presents an account of how many arts processes do demonstrate that care is realised through the activity of making and taking part in arts practices. However, it is also a proposal for greater attention to the caring possibilities of the arts in order that we might realise richer more life enhancing interhuman experiences. This is not caring or careful arts with social outcomes, but the integration of processes so that art making is simultaneously care taking.

Chapter 4 shifts focus into health and social care settings, examining Artful Care, or care practices that operate in an aesthetics register. This is not arts in health care contexts, but the 'art' of carers and the aesthetic experiences they enable through the relations they create with patients and others. The chapter draws on the history of health care professions use of aesthetic language in their outline of the knowledge and skills of nurses, by way of example, and examines the differences between what has been called 'the art of nursing' and the proposal here for an aesthetics of their care. The chapter then places the argument for care aesthetics alongside other related modes of analysis of care work, in particular the idea of *bodywork* and then the perspectives brought by concepts such as *affective* or *emotional labour*. The chapter explains how it borrows from these modes of analysis but also then differs from them. Chapter 4 is, in a sense, where an analysis of Grace as someone who creates exemplary care aesthetics experiences takes place.

The final chapter moves beyond the specific realms of the arts and health and social care, to explore how care aesthetics can be taken as a way of understanding interhuman relations in the everyday. It asks what would happen if we acted with attention to the aesthetics of our care for people in our communities and neighbourhoods, in our everyday engagements with them. This is not as an alternative site of care from the arts and health, but an acknowledgement that the boundaries between professional or vocational care, and that which we undertake in our daily routines or daily interactions, in fact borrow from each other. We draw on the skills and sensory practices from our professional lives to practice everyday care, and similarly, our professional lives are animated by how we are cared for by others or care for others in our everyday. The chapter takes several examples of responses to the Coronavirus pandemic to make the case that this particular care crisis in fact stimulated a range of care aesthetic responses, where the lines between art activities and care activities were blurred. While it is important to acknowledge the terrible outcomes from the pandemic, there were also cases where an artful practice of care was distributed beyond the formal settings and became a vital mode of engagement for an everyday solidarity between communities meeting the pressing demands of the crisis.

The book ends with some tentative suggestions as to where future care aesthetics research and practice might develop. It is acknowledged that the book is written from the context of the UK and a particular cultural and historical moment of care. It is not written by an author whose close friends need to leave their homes for care-related employment in distant countries; it is not written by someone who is paid to care or needs daily care to make full participation in everyday life possible. While I have been and am currently in a position where I care for others, and similarly in the past I have needed the care of others, the shape and feel of care aesthetics will ultimately be best explained by those who have an intimate connection to care, and the nuances of their care experiences will change dependent on multiple related factors. The claim here is that, while recognising the inequalities of international care economies, in many contexts care is experienced, often against all odds, for its intense warmth and beauty. The book's starting point is that we need to hold onto these moments, to value them, and champion those capacities that make this sensory richness more likely and more sustained. If too often our societies give recognition and status to the intrepid individualist who is rewarded for being carefree and careless, Care Aesthetics seeks to offer a space when mutual support in all its dynamism gets the focus and attention it so richly deserves. It is a book that seeks to give value to those artists of quality caring relations too often ignored. It is a book, to borrow again from Roger Robinson's poem, that gives space to G/grace.

Part I
Care Aesthetics

1

What is the *aesthetics* of care aesthetics?

Chapter 1 explains how *aesthetics* is being used in the concept care aesthetics. It borrows from a history of aesthetic theory, and contemporary uses of the word within the fields of socially engaged arts and health and social care. The approach is inevitably expansive to provide a definition that can include caring relations within its ambit. While this will be counter to some traditions of aesthetic theory, it is by no means exceptional. One of the opening statements of Bence Nanay's '*Aesthetics: A Very Short Introduction*' asserts that its scope is 'far wider than that of art' and in fact 'includes much of what we care about in life' (2019: 2). Answering the question *what is the aesthetics of care aesthetics*, therefore, starts from a broad interpretation that includes much that we care about and, in fact, as will be explained in the pages below, is helpful in understanding care itself.

The chapter opens with six vignettes. They are deliberately diverse in context and cover descriptions from both the arts and practices that are 'far wider than that of art'. They are presented here to illustrate the scope of care aesthetics, but also raise some of the issues that will recur throughout the book. They are not exemplars in the sense of presenting care aesthetics without problems. The ambition is that they suggest what care aesthetics refers to and what issues are raised by the term. Each presents questions: for example, about power, about caring labour, and about who determines what is understood as good or bad care. Those involved in applied theatre and the socially engaged arts will recognise the youth theatre rehearsal, and readers from health and social care will be familiar with the bathing example and debates about intimate bodywork. The COVID example is chosen to raise some of the issues that will be returned to across the work but specifically in Chapter 5. The 'axe' example is used to draw attention to the themes of hierarchies in value in art and craft practices and the debates about functionality and beauty. The pottery example is used to touch on similar

DOI: 10.4324/9781003260066-3

questions and then also as a nod to Japanese aesthetics which will feature later in this chapter. Reading each example invites attention to how experiences are crafted, how bodies interact, how the senses are engaged, and how people attend to each other. In taking care of a person, an object, or a process, and being taken care of within a particular context, they start to give shape to the ideas and concerns that *care aesthetics* seeks to capture.

Bathing

If you bathe an elderly relative, partner, or patient, you might start by considering the temperature of the water. You may dip your elbow to assess its warmth, and this could be as a technical check to assess the heat that is best for cleaning an older person's skin, or a more familiar one done to see if it was right for giving the maximum pleasure. Or maybe determining the difference between these two is impossible. Is warm water practical or does it just feel good? Then you might lift, support, or ease them into the water. With an aid or not depending on their mobility. If you physically lift them, even with a mechanical lift to help, you will have to exert yourself physically in the manoeuvre. You may hold an arm, touch a shoulder, or cup an elbow. They will hold you. This will be done with a balance between the firmness required to move someone, but the gentle precision to ensure that they are reassured that they will not tilt, rock, or shift too suddenly or painfully. You are likely to speak to them throughout the whole process. While the conversation at this time might be nothing to do with the bathing – an aside about other family members, personal interests, the weather, or mutual jokes about common interests – there will be a tone in the voice that seeks to attune to the movement of the other person and the moment at hand. The focus of your eyes will be important, even if done without self-awareness. You might be looking into their eyes, or avoiding them due to embarrassment, or noting the impediments in the environment. You might be watching them intently, trying to keep attention to the anxieties, or simple expressions of concern that might flicker across their face. And they too will choose words and tone – sometimes to reassure you that they are comfortable with what is happening, or to distract you from your concerns about their welfare. Once in the bath, you may leave them if that is their preference, and safety permits. Or you may stay awhile and help them wash. Or simply as company to chat about lives, loves, and everyday matters. If you do stay with them to wash them, you will choose cloth, soap, and then the position of your hand and the pressure it applies. You may wear gloves if this is a professional relationship but may not if you are caring for your own loved one. Your gentleness of touch will be related to your desire to fulfil the need for them to be, and to feel, clean and also the soothing feeling of being soaked with warm water. The bathing finished; your joint endeavour is over – to be repeated maybe at another time. It might have been slow, difficult, perhaps emotionally draining for both parties, or it might have been close, warm, and heartening. Or a mixture of all these.

Physiotherapy

When my friend Antoine Muvunyi had an operation on his shattered elbow in 2011, he needed nearly six months of physiotherapy during his recuperation. A bullet had entered his forearm and exited through his humerus above his elbow joint. His elbow had been resting out of the window of their van, and this particular shot wizzed along the side going clean in and out of his arm. In severing the nerve that runs over the tip of his elbow, and his elbow having been rebuilt with a lattice of metal plates, he had lost the feeling and most of the movement in his fingers. It was their gentle manipulation which was the focus of most of his post-operative therapy. When Antoine arrived in the UK, he had very little English, although as with many people in the Democratic Republic of the Congo, he had at least five other languages. His negotiation with his physiotherapist was therefore in a form of broken communication, and an intensity of touch and gaze. As she held his hand, he had to hold her in his eyes. One sense was tuned into the other, and as she pressed, twisted, and manipulated the joints, the grip of his stare shifted in strength as it indicated the pain that he was in. At certain points, he would suck deeply on the supply of gas and air, using his uninjured left hand to draw the mask to his face. And then drop it, with a nod to his therapist, who would then nod back and continue. There was a pattern of massage on the palm, fingers, and knuckles that used the rhythm of what appeared to be the rolling pain he was in, to intensify and ease off in turn. It was a toing and froing that seemed to be a physical dialogue that was attempting to pressure his hand back to life. And the touch, the tenderness, and the eye-ball-to-eye-ball trust appeared to give him the strength to commit to the process. He nodded and gave into her skill. It was executed with the dexterity and attention to detail of a true craftsperson: someone who had immense knowledge and a capacity to execute it in a way that adapted in response to the person who was in front of her. The quality of the relationship between them, build through touch and facial understanding, changed over the months as they seemed to develop a rhythm of call and response. The object of her craft was not an inanimate thing to be shaped, but a responsive and gradually responding part of Antoine's recovering body. An arm, and a hand, that would have been lost was returned to a level of function that meant Antoine could return to work back home in the DRC.

Hot water bottle

Shoji Hamada was designated a National Living Treasure in Japan in 1955, a first for pottery and also for crafts more broadly. He was a master potter known internationally for the simple, earthy pots he created and sold all over the world. Since his death in 1988, his workshops have been turned into a museum called the Mashiko Museum of Ceramic Art where visitors can see his collections and the studio in which he made his work. One of the most extraordinary demonstrations of his skills can be seen in a short, grainy black and white film from 1968 simply called *Shoji Hamada Pottery* where he demonstrates his use of the potters' wheel and the delicate manipulation of clay. Always steady, intricate, and constantly moving, he turns the wheel by hand and cups each finished item before delicately laying it to the side. In the process, we see his body, his fingers, and the wheel in constant motion and then the emerging clay pot extending and rising from his movements. It is difficult to understand how each touch on the clay makes it move in the way it does. Each small piece seems to have a smooth yet somewhat unfinished quality. The most extraordinary single item he makes in this film is the water bottle. He builds the piece over time, almost in waves, and it becomes many things in the viewers mind – a vase, a tea pot, a large urn. His hands, in the black and white film, seem at one with the clay, both controlling and determining the shape, but somehow responding to a form that is perhaps already implicit in the material. It is a caress, a gentle cajoling of the form from within the clay. Working on the water bottle, it is impossible to know what the shape will be, or to know if he knows the shape the clay would like. Towards the end of the process, he neatly brings the top of the large cylinder together practically closing the end but leaving a tiny hole. The smooth and perfectly rounded shape is lifted like a small animal off the wheel and then surprisingly rather than placing it on its flat end as would be expected, he lies it on its side, and it slumps. It almost breathes downwards into its new position. The side becomes the base and you hear a voice in English ask him what it is, and then the same voice announces that it is a hot water bottle.

The axe

There can be great pleasure in using an axe to cut wood. Maybe it is the feel of the handle, the delight in splitting a log in one go, the gleam of the sharp edge in the daylight, or the final achievement of a stack of almost uniform length firewood. And this is particularly the case when using an axe with a carved, perhaps ornate handle, made with the rich sheen of hard wood. Maybe the pleasure comes from the physical exertion, but it must also be the movement of the head with its high polish and unusual shape. And it is also the sharp crack from the splitting of wood so precise that it can be stacked in a wood store with neat ends making patterns with the other logs. There is the balance of the axe, the weight ratio between handle and head, that makes the task more efficient, but there is also significant pleasure in the sense of equilibrium. A *good* axe makes the time go by quicker, but there is also a losing of an awareness of time in the task. The wood is for burning, so while ornamental in the stack it is also necessary as a source of heat for the home. Every time you come to fetch some of your cut wood, there is a tiny moment of reluctance as you have to change the patterns in which it is piled. You might pause before a new bundle is stuffed into a basket, as the symmetrical rows of drying kindle are almost too beautiful to be used. If a photograph was taken of your wood pile, and then displayed in a gallery, the name of the photographer, and not yours, would be next to the image. The artistry would belong to the photograph, and not to your effort of careful, deliberate stacking. If your axe itself were displayed, there would be no name. Making axes, along with the many objects of everyday life, is the work of anonymous craftspeople. You need to photograph your axe to have your name alongside it. Or you need to curate the *rare axe exhibition* at a gallery, perhaps a folk-art museum, if your name is to be worthy of acknowledgement.

A youth theatre rehearsal

Young people hang off each other, seated in a circle as the director explains the final preparations for their performance. She has her hands out pushing the air down in a calming motion, expressing the need for the group to maintain focus, to keep relaxed and confident, in these final moments leading to a performance. She takes time to reassure, to catch eyes, and smile through the detailed notes on scenes and tiny moments of the play. The youth are on the floor, cross legged, sometimes lounging into each other, as forms of connection and mutual support, seem to hold them to a monumental task. A boy with red hair leans into a girl with braids. A large boy is hugged by a smaller one. The awkwardness of teen bodies seems to lock together as they attend to the director's words. They fire back concerns, comments, and underscores, which ripple around the circle, responded to by others, or quietened by the young woman director who also sits in the circle. The exceptional attention is new and not spontaneous in this group. They have built over many weeks a sense of connection across similarity in age but diversity of perspective and experience. New relations have been made, and identities morphed through the energy and tension required to realise the approaching performance. There have been multiple minor irritations, alliances, and disputes coalescing and then dispersing across the rehearsals and workshops. But now they protect the forthcoming public showing, and gut-filled belief in its importance, with a common sense of urgency and pride. It is all of theirs.

Balconies

In early April 2020, we gathered on our doorsteps to sing the Beatles song – 'With a little help from my friends'. A colleague posted an image of himself with amp and electric guitar doing his own garage (drive?) rock version with his neighbour up the street doing the bass line. This was the week after the first *clap for the carers*, when in the UK huge numbers came out of their front doors, or hung out from their windows, to clap, cheer, and bang pans to acknowledge the immense task of the National Health Service and other carers across the country. They had been putting their lives in danger, as they treated the terrible influx of very sick patients into the hospitals with COVID-19. We did not know then that we would still be locked down the following year, and much initial community solidarity was becoming strained by an incompetent government and a sense that applause was no substitute for properly funded health and social care. Our clapping was an echo of the videos that we had all seen circulating of Italians singing songs from their balconies, as they connected across courtyards during their long period of isolation. Images of men playing accordions, women bashing tambourines, and kids dancing led to a range of online and news outlet commentaries about resilience, community cohesion, and the role of creativity in adversity. They were both poignant and uplifting, yet also disturbing in how quickly a population could be isolated and restricted so drastically. These were the first documents of an artistic response to community-wide house arrest, and they became a touchstone of other responses as the weeks of lockdown continued. Being out of touch with your neighbours, friends, and family led to new ways of staying in touch. While much of this was online, in copious forms of domestic small screen performance, these acts of applause broke open our lockdown, to make links with our neighbours and other residents in our communities. Imperfect and not a substitute for decent protective clothing for nurses and health care staff, but an attempt at connection against the necessary isolation. Music and sound featured a lot in these examples as an activity that many could join in with, but also as something that carried across the air between people, when actual physical touch was prohibited. We all applauded, but also heard and felt the applause of others. Sound did not obey the rules of social distancing and was a way of connecting that also reminded us all of the disconnections that were being experienced.

Bathing and the feel of warm water. Massaging and receiving a massage. Gently turning clay into an object to ward off the cold. Enjoying the well-made axe. Holding onto peers as a performance is prepared. Singing across balconies to your neighbours. The argument here is that each of these describes an aesthetic experience. I hope to justify this claim, but to start I need to go backwards into a philosophical tradition, to find a point of departure that permits this inclusivity.

In her book *The Way of Love*, French philosopher Luce Irigaray makes a comment on the history of Western Philosophy which acts as an indictment of the focus of attention of the predominantly male writers. She suggests:

> The Western philosopher wonders very little about the relation of speaking between subjects. It is the relation between subject and object or a thing that he tried to say or to analyze, hardly caring about speaking to the other
> *(2002: 15)*.

Of course, this may be countered by drawing attention to the work of Martin Buber in his seminal work on the relation between 'I and Thou', or Emmanuel Levinas' concern for the ethical call of the *face of the other*. However, I want to accept the thrust of Irigaray's critique as it helps to draw attention to how Western *aesthetic* theory has, by and large, also *wondered very little* about the relations between subjects. For a chapter that seeks to lay out what the *aesthetics* in care aesthetics might refer to, this is a problem. In the 1990s, Irigaray undertook a research project analysing children's use of language and in particular the way they speak in the first person (see Hirsh and Olson, 1995). While the essentialism of her analysis might be questioned, her findings give more substance to the quotation above. In her research, she was focusing on the gendered use of the word *avec* – with. When asking children who or what they were playing *with*, the boys would nearly always refer to an object – I play *with* a truck, a toy, or a ball. When asking girls the same question, they would mention a person, often a friend. So, for them, it was – I play *with* Suzanne or *with* my sister. In a sweeping claim, drawing on what she saw as a fundamental linguistic difference, Irigaray shows how a foundational preoccupation with the relations between object and subject, objectivity and subjectivity, with the thingness of thing in front of you, is not the obvious and necessary focus of philosophical enquiry, but a peculiar one, particular in a large part to the speaking habits of men. Whether this is a sociological or psychological propensity is not for the analysis here, but the notion of different speech amongst men and women, will reappear as a trope in the early work on care ethics which is the subject of the next chapter. Transposing this to the focus of this chapter, it offers an explanation for a similar tendency in the field of aesthetics. If Western philosophy has to a certain extent focused on the relation between subject and object, then the sub field of aesthetics has also tended to focus on the objects in front of us, the paintings on the wall, or the play on the stage. Aesthetics as a field of enquiry has relied on an unquestioned orientation to things and not to *speaking with the other*. Questions of taste, of beauty, of the judgement of value or quality, of purpose, and of meaning, have been framed by an assumption, a type of unexamined common sense, that there is a thing in front of us and that our relation to that thing is the most important concern for aesthetic enquiry.

Irigaray makes us think again. For her, it is the person in front of us that is more important and our relation with that other, and other others, is central. *Hardly caring* about the other, is a particular gendered orientation that needs to shift to a new position where we are at least asking questions about what subject-to-subject attention might be. Irigaray's provocation is, therefore, the starting point of this chapter. If we are to ask how care might have an aesthetics, and if it does, what that aesthetics might consist of, we have to enlist this perspective, this orientation to the other, as the opening proposition. The first argument for the aesthetics of care aesthetics is, therefore, a challenge to an assumption as to what the 'avec' might refer. Rather than a sole focus on the contemplation of objects, whether still or moving, care aesthetics *cares profoundly* about speaking with, being with and working with another person, and other people.

Leaving the essentialism of Irigaray' claim that boys are 'avec' their toys, and girls are 'avec' their friends to one side for the moment, another reason her quotation is important for the discussion that follows, is that she does not identify 'The Western Philosopher' by name. She is making the general proposition that philosopher boys are focused on their toys. The un-naming is important here, because there is a tendency in accounts of *aesthetics* for them to consist of texts peppered with different names and accounts of their marginally different perspectives. While this chapter clearly draws from accounts of aesthetics in a largely Western philosophical literature, I want to avoid this tendency and instead explain the themes that are important for this particular account, without taking too much space allocating different perspectives to different original texts. I am, therefore, also borrowing from Irigaray in not over naming, but instead developing ideas and orientations that many different writers have offered. This includes the relations between people and between people and objects as touched on here, but also it will examine other important questions of aesthetics for making the case for an aesthetics of care. This includes issues of aesthetic theory and the philosophy of art, the notions of autonomy and heteronomy, function and beauty, aesthetic experience, social aesthetics and everyday life, and then concepts of sense and 'the sensory world'. The chapter will also include an examination of relationality, what are labelled 'proximal' and 'distal' senses, what is called here *in between* aesthetics, and the body and self-care. The final parts of the chapter, where there will be more sources referenced, will include a reflection on the importance of Japanese aesthetics. This acts as an acknowledgement that the problems I am outlining are located primarily in a Western tradition, but it is also to make the link more explicit between aesthetics and ethics which emerges from within a certain Japanese tradition, which in turn sets up the discussion of Chapter 2.

The chapter will use the opening vignettes to illustrate points made throughout. As I wrote above, these are not exemplary cases of care aesthetics, rather a selection that help reflect on its range and potential points of contact. The chapter is seeking to claim that human caring, and in particular human-to-human caring, is a reasonable focus for aesthetic theory. The starting point, as discussed above, is that the *aesthetics* of care aesthetics is interested in the relations between people, challenging a presumed *avec* the object with an *avec* that includes others (and does not reject objects entirely as will be explained below). We need an understanding of aesthetics that can account for the craft of those relations, how they exercise power or collaboration, how they enact hierarchies or equalities, and how they have a sensation of delight or pain. Importantly, aesthetics can be used as a classificatory category which might include the negative or unpleasant, but it is often used in an honorific sense, where being commended for an *aesthetic* implies a positive quality. This distinction, between classificatory or descriptive and honorific or evaluative, will be developed below.

While relations with the other have become a subject of aesthetics more recently, Irigaray's distinction presented here is meant as a reorientation and not a complete disavowal of relations to objects. As can be seen from the opening vignettes, there are accounts of relations between people, and relations to objects. The account of the Japanese potter or the beautifully crafted axe is crucial to show that objects, and care for them, will be an important element of care aesthetics and this will be dealt with in more detail later. The point to emphasise is that while objects can become part of the other-regarding focus of care aesthetics, the *picture on the wall*, or the toys in the hands of boys, are rejected as the solitary point of departure. This is a familiar claim if we extend our focus beyond *Western* aesthetics to Indigenous craft traditions documented by writers such as Robin Wall Kimmerer (2013) or the African aesthetic traditions discussed by Kwame Anthony Appiah (1997). We need to start caring about the speaking other, in Irigaray's words, and that relation is a vital emphasis for a relational caring aesthetics, but one that will not reject the care we take of the objects in our lives.

Aisthesis

The word aesthetics derives from the Greek *aisthesis* meaning sensory perception and was originally used to make a distinction from intellectual or cognitive perception. We might today refer to this as *embodied sensory perception* but the point to emphasis is that aesthetics as a field does not start as the study of art, but from sensory experience, of which art may be a significant part. Art may produce an aesthetic experience (and more about *experience* below) but it is not the only human activity or natural phenomenon that does so. Care aesthetics is, therefore, not using aesthetics as a synonym for art. A study of aesthetics is not the same as the philosophy of art, and while there are strong relationships between art and aesthetics, to make the case that the relations between people can be understood aesthetically, the point of their difference has to be emphasised. Many aspects of life have an aesthetic quality and holding onto an expansive and inclusive definition helps us show the diversity of the aesthetic experiences of our different lives. The common assumption that aesthetics means philosophy of art results in art becoming the focus for commentary on the subject rather than the other ways that aesthetic experience and aesthetic pleasure is realised in different contexts. This is important because for care aesthetics as a concept to work, it needs to question the art-centric orientation where from art comes aesthetics and not the other way around. It accepts that artists, and the galleries, theatres and museums where their work is displayed, create aesthetic experiences, but they are not its sole purveyors.

In focusing on aesthetics, rather than that subset which is the visual, creative, and performing arts, there is a challenge to the tendency for aesthetic debates to illustrate their arguments only through examples of artistic work. Even those accounts which accept the general position that aesthetics as sensory perception and experience occurs in a multitude of contexts, often then revert to analysing art projects or artists. Of course, aesthetic experiences created through artistic practice or engagement might be particularly profound but the purpose here is to challenge the automatic hierarchy in aesthetic theory that assumes that the arts and artists can claim that they are the only architects of a certain type of heightened sensory experience. From the vignettes, singing from the balcony in the particular context of COVID-19 is an aesthetic experience for those singing and those listening, but it is not because it used an art form that it can make this claim. Rather it is the contours of that sensory experience within particularly difficult moment of time, that made it so. The argument here is that singing from a balcony *and* bathing an elder both deserve attention for their aesthetics, and one is not prioritised for analysis or approval because it exists in the register of what has traditionally been called 'the arts'.

What follows from the assertion that the arts are a component part of the field of aesthetics and not its exemplar or synonym, is that the arts should not be given a position of greater significance solely because of their existence as the arts. Some artistic endeavour might produce pleasurable and meaningful experiences, but this does not mean that it should automatically be given priority for analysis or attention. This expansiveness, attending to multiple possible sources for aesthetic experience more equally, connects to one of the dominant debates within aesthetic theory and is important for the claim that care can be considered for its aesthetic properties. This is the relationship between autonomy and heteronomy in aesthetic theory. The former presents aesthetics, and specifically the arts as an aesthetic activity, as an independent area of practice, separate from other areas of social life. The latter asserts that aesthetic experiences, and arts practices that create them, are properly understood as interdependent, and intricately embedded within the world. The argument for autonomy stretches from a belief that art should be judged on its own terms and not by standards or values linked to other areas, to a belief that an independent artistic realm is a necessary place of freedom apart from the social constraints of the everyday. The arguments for autonomy are primarily focused on arts practices and less on the more expansive definition of aesthetics used here and can be summarised in the over neat maxim of *arts for art's sake*. Autonomy seeks to delineate an aesthetic realm that values an appreciation of beauty that while meaningful has no meaning that points to a purpose beyond the art itself. Similarly, these arguments include the more radical ambition for the arts to provide a space that can create transformative experiences that cannot be captured by a market economy based on the designation of monetary value and exchange. A claim for artistic autonomy has been a feature of aesthetic theory from Kant, through Marcuse and Adorno, and reappears in diverse writers some seeking to conserve the special place for the fine arts, and others seeking to validate the radical disruption enabled by avant-garde arts practices. While there are important lessons to be learnt from the tradition of valuing or demanding artistic autonomy, by making the case for care to be considered aesthetically, there is an axiomatic critique of the insistence that the aesthetic realm is autonomous. If the work of the physiotherapist treating my friend and the bathing of an elder relative have aesthetic properties, there must be a claim that aesthetics is embedded in a multitude of activities that are part of our daily routines. This would, therefore, imply that care aesthetics is committed to an alternative, more heteronomous view.

Heteronomy suggests that aesthetic experiences are firmly of the world and imbricated in diverse social practices. They borrow from values and concepts from across our life worlds in a promiscuous way so that to talk of an independent artistic sphere makes little sense. If aesthetic experience is a human experience, even if related to the appreciation of fine art, it is difficult to insist that it is separate from the world in which it takes place. A heteronomous perspective points to what Arnold Berleant has called *social aesthetics* (2011) where the arts in particular, and their differentiation into categories, forms, and genres, are products of particular histories and geographies and not discrete phenomena. The argument here is that the concept of autonomy itself is a social product, a gradual accretion of practices and theories seeking out definition and distinction for a particular capacity, largely related to the appreciation of visual art. An account of aesthetics which wills the artist to have an independent responsibility, whether for creating purposeless beauty or liminal transformational experiences, is itself a product of a peculiar set of historical circumstances. The theory of aesthetic autonomy is, thus, an aspiration and value-based claim and not a description of the world as it is. Even if the aesthetic experience is hard to explain, perhaps overwhelming and seemingly beyond words, the argument here insists it is still part of a particular body or groups of bodies, whose presence in space belongs concretely to a certain social world. If that experience struggles to fit conceptually into frameworks that are familiar, and perhaps even feels unattached to any obvious social purpose, it is still of a time, in a place, and affective within a particular set of physical constraints. Learning from theories of autonomy can help us appreciate how aesthetics experiences might take us outside a certain social moment, but to extend this to say that aesthetics operates outside the parameters of the social, in its own distinct realm, fails to recognise that demands for artistic independence are themselves part of a particular, not universal, social history.

Care aesthetics, therefore, starts from heteronomy, because a claim that care can be an aesthetic experience is de facto locating aesthetics within social practices and daily life. It is an argument for an aesthetics embedded in and related to multiple people and contexts of the social world and not independent of them. Care aesthetics proposes an aesthetics that demonstrates an interdependence, structured through multiple subjects and practices. This aesthetics must be of and between the bodies, objects, and environments of the world. This, of course, does not mean that we cannot try to identify the specific elements of an aesthetic experience and focus on these for the sensations or pleasures they provoke. For example, I can listen to the singing of the balcony and concentrate on its timbre, rhythm, choice of form, and resonance but my argument here is that these are first intricately connected to the immediate context in which they are experienced, and second, this acknowledgement of the wider context does not diminish my appreciation of them. In fact, the strain of the voice becomes more moving because I know the man is trying to project it to a balcony on the other side of the street. The exuberance with which he sings is heightened by the sight of a woman and child dancing on another balcony. It is how his singing is embedded in the immediate social context and is related to other acts of movement and music, that extends rather than weakens my sensory perception of it. My knowledge that these individuals are locked down in a community that at the time was facing the worse of the COVID-19 crisis, does not diminish the aesthetics of these musical performances but adds to their weight. A social context, here the pandemic, magnifies the powerful quality of the song and does not restrain it by making it dependent on concepts, such as social cohesion or community solidarity.

The emphasis in care aesthetics, therefore, is one of an aesthetic interdependence, of being bound within a social context in which a practice finds itself. Being caught in this way is not a submission to constraint, somehow a restriction of aesthetic and arts practices so that they have no freedom. It is a willing recognition of the integrated position of aesthetic experience, and not a normative announcement that the arts must submit. This notion of interdependence will be taken up in the second chapter as it strongly links to the field of care ethics, but here it is taken as a realistic account of the way aesthetic experience is located within our lives. In comparing the axe in my hand as I chop wood, and the axe displayed in the museum, I do not compare heteronomy with autonomy. Both *uses* have dependencies and contexts that feed into the appreciation of the beauty or general experience of that axe. While I will discuss the fact that the axe in my hand is appreciated with a different set of senses from those that *view* the axe in the museum below, to develop the idea of interdependence it is important to focus on that use. Rather than dismissing the *function* of that object from a discussion of aesthetics, I want to develop the notion of what will be called here *purposeful beauty*.

Purposeful beauty

The notion of purpose is a subset of the debates between autonomy and heteronomy in the history of aesthetics, whereby an appeal beyond the aesthetics of the art, to a function that meets a need extraneous to it, is either disparaged or welcomed. A classic statement of this debate can be found in the book by Glenn Parsons and Allen Carlson called *Functional Beauty* (2008). When equipment, tools, or objects with clear purposes are dismissed as obviously not part of the world of aesthetics, we see a reification of objects that have no apparent tool-like function. In the case for autonomy, art is valued for its self-sufficiency, appealing to taste, or affective response without an external referent. In fact, however, the denial of purpose actually hides implicit function, which is the delineation of the art world itself: the creation of a realm of distinction. Art's purpose is to make itself distinct as art. Disparaging function thus produces the seemingly purposeless art world that draws on its appeal to men and women of a certain taste and ability to distinguish it. An alternative approach that focuses instead on aesthetic experiences would allow our understanding of purpose to become richer and more differentiated. Welcoming diverse *purposes* in fact expands the textures and affects of an aesthetic experience and the task should perhaps be to imagine a multitude of connections and possible relations to the social world, emanating from a particular experience. The warm water in a bath for yourself, for your children, or for an elderly relative, soothes the skin, cleans the body, and produces a sense of relaxation or joy (a theme taken up in the performance work of Adrian Howells in Chapter 3). Imagining the extended sensations from the moment does not sully a somehow pure, self-sufficient aesthetic, but rather it enriches it. The argument here is that this is the same for a picture on a wall, for the design of an axe head, and for the touch of the physiotherapist.

One important question for care aesthetics that emerges from this approach is whether there is a boundary between beauty and purpose. At what point does attention to function end and attention to aesthetics begin and can we in fact delineate the purely aesthetic from the purely purpose-related? As I design the axe does the ornamental carving of the handle operate separately from my design of its grip or balance. When are those criss-cross groves cut solely to prevent slipping and when does enjoyment of their delicate symmetry begin? As the physiotherapist was massaging my colleague's hand, could we make a distinction between the tenderness that was clinically necessary and that which was *a touch even more tender* than it needed to be? The argument here is that we should not see this as a continuum from purpose to beauty. This would assume that I first make a functional axe and then decorate its handle as an afterthought. The proposal here is that when the potter manipulates the clay to create the water bottle, we cannot draw a neat line to distinguish the moment the clay is smooth *enough* for the shape to function to hold warm water, and when it is perfected beyond any conceivable necessity. It could be argued that much Japanese craft ware plays exactly with this boundary. Purpose and beauty rather roll back and forth between each other, looping one apparently aesthetic decision into a functional one, and a functional adjustment into an aesthetic one. For an aesthetics of care, improving the touch, the tenderness, the quality of the hold, and the warmth of the regard, wraps function into quality in a way to make one dependent on the other, and mutually reinforcing of the other. So, as I hold a child's hand to cross the road, the security I and they might feel is in the tenderness *and* firmness of the grip, giving an experience of attentive calm and confidence in getting us both across the road safely. It is not mere secure grip; it is not just an act of tenderness. Heidegger famously complained that equipment was *half a thing,* or *half an artwork,* and my response is that in fact the beautifully purposeful *thing* can be twice an art work, doubled in its reach and significance.

Proximal and distal senses

For this argument to work, there is an important element of aesthetics that I have been drawing on here but not commenting on explicitly. This is the difference between proximal and distal senses and how within a particular tradition of aesthetic theory, the distal senses of sight and hearing are valued above those more immediate senses of touch, smell, and taste. If distal senses remain the primary concern, it leads to attention in aesthetic theory being only given to the objects in front of us, or the sounds we hear, and it means the discussion will be focused upon what capacities we bring to our appreciation or understanding of those things. When distal senses take primacy, when there is a tendency for the contemplative to be valued over and above other means of engaging with the world, the starting point for aesthetic debate becomes relative detachment. Proximal senses on the other hand, are those that are closer to the body, where we are kinaesthetically involved with that which surrounds us or with those whose lives we share. In mentioning this distinction, the point is not to dismiss the distal in favour of the proximal but to note that aesthetic experience should be valued for the somatic engagement it makes with our whole body which includes the full range of human sense making. Sole attention to sight means that aesthetics becomes the study of ocular perception and how we might stand back and reflect on what we behold. A fulsome, inclusive somatic approach means we start to focus on how we are involved in the moment, not just as witnesses, but as engaged participants.

The orientation endorsed here is one that shifts the narrow focus on aesthetics as the study of art to a broader exploration of embodied experience. This means we do not only consider a thing or person in front of us, primarily using our sight to reflect on their attributes. Instead, we broaden our concern to a practice of somatic attention where all elements of the aesthetic moment are considered as a whole. We attend to the object as a maker; we attend to another as carer; we attend to the moment as recipient of the attention of others. In the same way that there is no separate aesthetic sphere that operates under its own rules, out-side society, here the proposition is that there is aesthetic experience in which we are all part, rather than a neat boundary between a critic and the art they contemplate. These distinctions suggest that aesthetic experience is not a tangi-ble thing, but an activity. It is about a doing, a moving through the moment, in which a body in motion is somatically engaged with its surroundings and how it understands those surroundings through that immersion within them. Rather than a hierarchy of sense-based perception, which traditionally places *standing outside and watching* as the activity that through which we create insight, we have awareness developed through all the senses. Aesthetics is not merely the activity of the critic standing in front of your wood stack and reflecting on its symme-try, or the art aficionado commenting on the contours of the pot, but it occurs in the making, touching, smelling, and observing of those things. Aesthetics in care aesthetics needs a shift from contemplation as its primary mode to one of attending, not only in the sense of waiting alongside, but in terms of *attending in the moment*. This demands a certain absorption in the act as it unfolds, a quality of presence, and not the distilling of the activity to single sensory engagement. While we might attend to an image in front of us, attention here is meant more as the full-bodied involvement in an act. This orientation means that the starting point is not in prioritising the person who can comment on the quality of the shine of a wooden floor, but might also start with the skill, movement, and care of the cleaner who polished it in the first place (this point is taken up again in the account of the artist, Mierle Laderman Ukeles, in Chapter 3).

This focus challenges an orientation for aesthetic enquiry that assumes the observer, or the witness, are the exemplary purveyors of understanding, or the primary perspective makers for the field. Both the histories of Western aesthetics and art criticism have tended to be based on this default position because the writers are ultimately commenting on their experience of seeing visual art, visiting the theatre, or hearing music as audience members. Their point of access to the experience is assumed as the natural point of view from which our understanding of aesthetics emanates. We need to think instead of aesthetic experience as a total, multifaceted unfolding of an action. This would mean that the act of the witness is but one element of aesthetic appreciation. A broader approach is that we are all actors in aesthetic experiences, bringing them to life through our visceral involvement in them.

In between

In suggesting that distal and proximal senses taken together produce aesthetic experience, whether for maker, viewer, or participant, there is a danger if we only see the experience as the embodied sensations belonging to a single individual. Since Hume's work on taste and Kant's on beauty, there has been a broader acceptance that beauty is not in the object but in the aesthetic sensations experienced by the beholder. However, as pointed out above, this relies on a dyad of person and object, when the aim here is to develop an aesthetics that might respond to person to person, or inter-group experiences. Moving away from a purely visual relation between subject and its object, to the demand that we think of somatic relations in aesthetics, means that we should avoid psychologising aesthetic experience as the properties of the solitary person as she or he contemplates an external thing, and instead propose that it is a property that extends beyond and between bodies in action. It is evoked in moments between people as they engage with each other in diverse, sometimes artistic activities. Dancing together creates an aesthetic experience that flows across bodies in space and time. This does not mean it is the same experience for each person dancing, but there are sensations of touch and being touched, that emerge and are diffused between them. This is acknowledged by dance scholar Fiona Bannon when she explains her interest in 'what goes on between people in the creation and performance of particular works' (2018: 126). There is an *in between* aesthetics, that cannot be isolated to one part of a total experience. The person bathing a relative and the person being bathed by a relative will have an experience that is differentiated by their personal life experiences, but also somewhat in common shifting in, out, and between their bodies as they move through the process. Of course, the objects involved will also enhance or diminish the quality of this experience, as the bath, the water, grab bars, or lifting devices, contribute to the feelings evoked. *In between* aesthetics is important for thinking about care to ensure that the focus is not about the experience of one element of a complex interaction between people, either in pairs of carer and cared for, or in wider networks of social care.

On one level, this understanding of aesthetics has a small scale or intimate character. In mentioning dance above, I was implicitly suggesting that it is the touch between the dancers that permits the experience to have this *in between* quality. A dancer holds the hands of their partner, or draws another body close, and while individual abandon is of course a feature of many dance cultures, the companionship of much dance is a central feature for both participants and observers. The lift, and the skill *and* care demonstrated by its execution, is central to its affect (and these points are developed further in Chapter 3). This connects to the opening examples where the touch between people and the touch of objects was a key trope. In fact, even the clapping for the NHS and the singing from balconies were partly embodied responses to the absence of touch forced by social distancing at that time. The young people in the circle were held in the eyes of the youth theatre director as they held onto each other. In many ways skin-to-skin moments are exemplars of the *in between aesthetics* of care aesthetics because you cannot determine exactly where the experience lies, as all are simultaneously touching others and being touched by them. The experience both starts within the body and is felt from without. This register for care aesthetics, therefore, borrowing from the phenomenology of Merleau-Ponty (2013), means that we are concerned with the craft of the intimate, or an *art of touch*. This includes a range of practices such as massage, breast feeding, holding hands, physiotherapy, bathing, and dance training. These are micro moments, often of everyday life, that have too rarely been considered for their aesthetic qualities (and a particular focus on the everyday will be developed in Chapter 5). Of course, it is important to note here, and this is something that will be discussed in the following chapter, that in working in intimate relations we are also concerned with the dangers of touch, where it can be abusive or non-consensual. The aesthetics of many of these intimacies might be drawn to our attention because of their gentleness and quality of tenderness, and also care aesthetics will be concerned with the opposite, where they are ugly and cruel.

To claim that the sensation from an aesthetic experience flows between people and is felt through the qualities of attention different people bring to it, there is also a social model rather than an individualistic model of aesthetics being proposed. Even at the intimate level, it has a social element in that it is in the register of *with*, or the convivial. The social character of care aesthetics is crucial and in many ways proposing an aesthetics of our social relationships is inherent in the ambition of the term. This will also be discussed below in a critique of the individualistic focus of body care that is part of the 'somaesthetics' movement. However, for now it is important to acknowledge that care aesthetics is a form of 'social aesthetics' (Berleant, 2011: 772), but it seeks to emphasise the relations between people at its centre, and in addition, to suggest that it is the potential of aesthetics to be a means of nourishing relations between people across social contexts that is its main focus. If the social suggests a form of being in community, the aim is to emphasise, returning to Irigaray, an aesthetics of being *with* community. So, while it will be important to focus on the intimate qualities of care aesthetics, this broader social orientation suggests that care aesthetics has a more expansive concern for social arrangements, the structures of organisations and networks of interhuman relations of a greater scale.

Aesthetic experience

Throughout the chapter, I have referred to *aesthetic experience* and I want now to turn to why this phrase is central to a proposal for care aesthetics more squarely. This will then lead to considering the importance of the everyday in care aesthetic theory and the notion of a sensible world. First experience is used as the main descriptor of the aesthetic moment to distinguish it from the more traditional concern for the contemplation of an object. In the ambition to enlarge the scope for aesthetics beyond the arts, perhaps primarily associated with the Pragmatist philosophical movement in the US (Dewey, 2005), it was seen as a way of drawing attention to the flow of life, with humans involved in daily interactions with each other and the natural world. Experience is the sensory immersion in the world around us, and the ordering of those sensations through different flows of affect, perception, and cognition. There is both the general flow of experience, perhaps routine, habitual, and unremarked, and then experiences that stand out from that flow as somewhat heightened or special. The degree to which an experience takes the form of a unified entity beyond the mundane, is determined by a multitude of factors that rely on the interpersonal, cultural, historical, and the socially situated. An aesthetic experience is most frequently identified when a moment has a degree of sensory affect and strength of felt engagement. The distinction between daily mundane experience, which still must be a series of sensory relations with the people and world around us, and a heightened experience that becomes perceived as memorable or worthy of note, is not fixed and predictable. Exceptional aesthetic experiences have no cultural universality or hierarchy of worth. Also, it is wrong to see them as always of a certain scale or complexity. The making of a pot can become a marked moment in one's daily life, as could be attending the first night of a youth theatre show in which your child has a lead part. For an experience to be aesthetic experience, it seems to need a certain structure, an enhanced sense of crafted intent, a particular stimulus of embodied response or affective involvement, and a certain stand out feature which engages with some or all our senses in a way that shifts them from their usual axis. It might not alter the everyday but extend and enhance it. This can be a mere flicker of unusual attention, or an occurrence that shakes you to your very core.

Above I am describing a flow of daily life, which is itself a series of overlapping experiences, that then become heightened, expanded, or somewhat charged with a different feeling. It is both an interruption to a routine movement through the day but also maybe an extension of its existing rhythm. My emphasis here is firstly that we should not create a hierarchy of experiences to dictate which are worthy of the category aesthetic and a rejection of the assumption that the arts are the only means to produce them. Also, there must be a challenge of the idea that it takes a certain type of person to have aesthetic experiences and that they need a prescribed form of preparation and training in order to recognise or appreciate them. There are multiple different aesthetics experiences which for different individuals and groups are meaningful to different degrees, but one group has no right to assume their propensity for that experience is somehow more noble or worthy than others. And it is not a matter that exposure to the aesthetics experiences of one group, will make another group understand or appreciate the value of them. Most communities have lives with complex aesthetic experiences of different intensities, and the emphasis here is that it is opening up opportunities for meaningful and life-enhancing aesthetic experiences which is more important than the aesthetic, and in particular artistic, forms of which they are composed.

One of the debates here is the difference between an everyday experience and a 'special' or heightened one. This concern is connected to the field of *everyday aesthetics*, most famously outlined in the work of Yuriko Saito (2008, 2017). If we have a humdrum, everyday life which is perhaps expanded or heightened by rarer discrete moments of aesthetic experience, which are distinguished from our daily routines at whatever scale they exist in, where does the everyday end and the aesthetic experience begin? For care aesthetics, this is important because it is asking when does an act of caring become an aesthetic experience and if there is such a thing as a non-aesthetic experience of care. Two of the most respected commentators on everyday aesthetics have differences of opinion here. Richard Shusterman, drawing on Dewey, has articulated a vision of aesthetics experience that is distinct from the flow of daily routine, and in fact is distinguished from its boring or humdrum nature (2012). His view is that the category of aesthetic experience to be meaningful needs to be composed of moments that jump out from the routine, to give new, less familiar, sensory pleasures. Saito, on the other hand, seeks to emphasise how even those so-called dull routines have an aesthetic quality. Doing the laundry, washing clothes, and feeding the children involve, from her perspective, multiple aesthetic decisions, and micro aesthetic experiences. There is something valuable in both sides of this debate. The emphasis here is to argue that aesthetic experiences can exist in multiple sites, multiple registers, and at vastly different scales. However, by using the term *aesthetic experience*, it does point to moments that have a certain sensory stimulation and unusual quality that involve and prompt a particular type of attention. There will be a perfunctory way that I could bathe a relative, dance with a partner, or throw a pot. At a very basic level, these still have an aesthetics (which is where I agree with Saito). But in presenting a phrase like *care aesthetics*, I am suggesting a scale, perhaps degree of attention, that must be searching for a quality that extends the diminished sensory register within which much of life, and so much care, is executed. Settling on whether the aesthetic experience is part of our everyday lives or whether it presents those heightened moments that are exceptions to that everydayness, is in effect a decision to use care aesthetics as a descriptive or normative term (or classificatory or honorific as mentioned above). Acknowledging that it can be used in both ways (and more will be said about this later) is why I shift between the two positions here. Everyday acts of care can be small-scale aesthetic experiences, but in attending to the craft and sensory richness of that care, *aesthetic experience* as a term can also be useful as a way of indicating a particularly heightened one.

As a way of thinking through care aesthetics as it relates to the everyday, another term to consider is the notion of how we exist within a certain sensory world. While borrowing from Rancière's *sensorium* or *distribution of the sensible* (2004), and even early Marx's interest in 'practical human-sensuous activity' (Miles, 2011: 24), I will use this in a slightly different way. Here, it refers to the organisation of sensory perception across the field of our experience, and embeddedness of the body in interconnected sensory schemas. A given time and context will be shaped by different forms of sensory expression and engagement, through which humans will receive and produce different sensory stimuli. The contours, waves, and flows, of this sensory world shift across time, cultural context, and coalesce in smaller distinctive sub-practices. We are not *in* a sensory world, somehow determined by it and pulled along in an unforgiving sensory vortex where we feel, hear, or see as we are required. We are more *of* a sensory world, producing it through our actions, and produced by it as the sense acts of others interact with our affective lives. This is, therefore, connected to the concept of *habitus* from Bourdieu, indicating the ingrained dispositions of our bodies, and the way they shape how we perceive the social world (1977). A historical period's sensory world will have multiple culturally and technologically specific sensory norms, which would be strange to people outside that moment. This is also true geographically, with diverse sensory worlds of distinct and yet interconnected cultures. We also live in worlds with certain dominant and sub-dominant sensory patterns that overlap, co-exist, and contend which each other. There will be sensory micro worlds that borrow some aspects from others, while maintaining a degree of unique sensory practice. Then there will be a simultaneity of sense registers that operate seemingly with their own norms, in spite of other ways of living. And then there will be others that seek to dominate, actively seeking to overwhelm, or more insidiously gradually overload the sensory capacities of certain less powerful sensory schemas. While there is likely to be within any particular society, a certain broadly distinguishable 'perceptual commons' (Berleant, 2011: 10), one important argument here is that small-scale, sensory schemas exist within the tiniest of sub-groups, geographical boundaries, and practice communities. To connect this back to the focus on aesthetics, this could be the aesthetic experiences that pertain to a particular group of artistic practices and the felt responses of those that experience them. So, there might be a sensory sub-world for opera lovers, which exist in their particular expectations of aural and visual experience, that are on the one hand somewhat unique, but then connected with other broader sensory worlds linked to certain communities of class or geographic region. Similarly, there will be a sensory sub-world of physiotherapists, who have particular expectations of touch which mark out a set of sense expectations that both connect and compete with wider norms in any given society.

If Saito in the case I made above sees everyday aesthetics as relevant to the humdrum daily activities and not the exceptional, I would argue she is presenting aesthetics as a synonym for the sensory world which we all experience and inhabit. I prefer to present her version of everyday aesthetics as an account of the sensory world outlined above, because it seeks to capture a terrain of activity and response, that we all live through. In addition, in presenting bodily sensory engagements with the world around us as the overriding context for everyday aesthetic experiences, it allows us to acknowledge the differences and stratifications that exist within them. A sensory world is one where preferences and expectations can exclude and create damaging hierarchies of worth. *Care aesthetics* is a proposal that our sensory world is delineated by the feelings executed in the caring relations between individuals and groups, but it is also suggesting that the shape of those sensory schemas can diminish as well as enable human flourishing. To be a sensory world, therefore by definition, it must also be able to desensitise and anaesthetise. While I prefer not to use *regime* for the sensory world, because it suggests some higher power outside of the networks of bodies that maintain that world, it is useful for its suggestion of the power involved in any sensory configuration. Sensory worlds are *maintained* and that may be through consent, and equally through constraint. The quietness of children in certain Victorian households was a sensory micro world in this sense. The clapping for the NHS during the coronavirus outbreak, was partly a minor key intervention in a sensory world that had been radically reshaped by new sensory norms. The degree to which we can intervene in small or large sensory worlds is, of course, a point for debate. The issue to stay with though, is that we are immersed in contexts which shape a range of sensory, or Saito would say aesthetic experiences, of different degrees of intensity or note. My deviation from Saito would be to suggest that in the flows of sensations, positive, negative, and indifferent, that we experience from our waking moment, we do need to point to aspects of those experiences when they have a certain quality of form, intensity of feeling, or emotional affect. I would not want to deny the possibility that many activities that some might disparage do present qualities of these types, but still feel it important to focus attention on those of a particular intensity. We may be bathed, but only exceptionally note when a particular sense of connection is apparent. We may chop wood, but only at certain moments marvel at the beauty of the axe. We may be surrounded by countless sounds, but be particularly moved, or even overwhelmed by the singing of a person close to us. The sensory world is thus the ferment of our aesthetic experiences but not directly synonymous with it.

Analysis of the shape of our sensory worlds, from the broadest to the smallest schemas in which we operate in our homes, workplaces, religious communities, or social groups, is vital for any discussion of the aesthetics of care aesthetics. It draws attention to the aesthetic experiences permitted by or resistant to expectation and custom within these different formations. As mentioned above, this raises questions as to the way a sensory world changes and by what mechanism. The contours of this debate can be seen in elitist discussions of appropriate behaviour in cultural events, for example, whether you can clap between the movements in a symphony without social disapproval. Similarly, it is notable in anthropological accounts of generational changes in bodily behaviour such as in the bowing culture in Japan (Tahhan, 2014) or in the role of public hand holding between same sex couples and campaigns to counter the discrimination faced by them. The backdrop to these discussions, particularly within the socially engaged arts, is the broad debate as to whether a given sensory world changes through deliberate human aesthetic activity. The perspective to be developed in Care Aesthetics is to question the boundary between an interventionist, perhaps activist response to this question and an ameliorative or gradualist one. We both simultaneously live within and respond to our sensory worlds, and the intensity of our sensory activities, or perhaps the craft brought to our aesthetic experiences is always varied and differentiated. A person paid to care who determinedly ensures the quality of the service she supplies in spite of the constraints faced might see herself as intervening in the cruelties of care, or might see it as her own sensory, affective response that simply aims for a slight improvement in the circumstances. The point to emphasise is that her ambition might shift across different circumstances, but we should recognise the minor and major efforts people make within the sensory worlds within which they operate. They should be valued if and where they are seeking some degree of transformation in the way a particular sensory scheme nourishes or sustains lives and makes relations between them more equitable.

A sensory world is made of multiple cross-connecting relations, between people and people, people and objects and between people and the natural world. Aesthetic experiences, in those marginally or intensively heightened moments of the everyday, are embedded in and emerge from these relations. As the opening examples suggest, it might be in the relation between the bather and the bathed, the patient and his physiotherapist, but also in the potter and his clay, or the wood chopper and her or his axe. These relations are the source of the *in between* discussed above, or the *avec* of Irigaray. While I focused on one-to-one relations in these examples, it is important to consider networks of relations between multiple points as the weave of a sensory world, and the sustaining framework for the aesthetic experiences that connect through our lives. The aesthetics here is found in the bonding of the links between people, those subtle bodily inflections that produce affection and recognition. The hyper-organised and crafted stage show maximised for the affective overload of an audience, is a version of this at a particular scale. The gentle welcome by a host, with the carefully considered body movements and hand gestures chosen to put a guest at ease, is an example at a more modest scale. The aesthetics here is not in the appreciation post hoc, but the sensory experience of being in relation to someone or something, or across a multitude of people and things across a distinct moment. This is why for youth theatre the rehearsal, the notes session, and the final performance are all part of the aesthetic experience. While it is impossible to locate the beginning and end of it precisely, it is in the awareness of a certain intensity in a series of relationships within a certain stretch of time that marks it out. And it marks out one that is likely to prompt the demand to form more, or hope for more, relations of a similar quality and intensity.

Self-fashioning

In focusing here on relations, and the importance of relations to any theory of aesthetics that insists that care between people can institute an aesthetic experience, there is one relation on which I have so far not commented. This is one that is important both for the field of aesthetics and also for care, and while I have been avoiding commentary too directly on different theorists here, the main location comes from the field called *somaesthetics* – a term coined by pragmatist philosopher Richard Shusterman. This is an area of practice and study that asserts the need to focus on our soma, our sensing and perceiving body, and in particular 'to give the body more careful aesthetic attention' (Shusterman, 2012: 6). The relation here is, therefore, not to someone other, but to the self and particularly the care for the self in programmes of 'self-fashioning' (Schusterman, 2000: 138). Self-care as a form of bodily focused aesthetics is perhaps the most significant area of aesthetic theory and practice where care and aesthetics are explicitly connected. There is a diversity of forms and practices that are part of this aesthetic relation to the self, including bodily adornment, such as tattoos, painting nails, hairstyling and facials, as well as body building and plastic surgery. It can mean adding to the body or enhancing the performance of the body. It can be an instant result of a fleeting activity or a sustained process over many years. It can draw on aesthetic ideals of the beautiful from rapidly changing assumptions about correct shape and attributes of the body, as well as self-care traditions drawn from practices with long cultural histories. Various martial arts, for example, and their diverse means of disciplining the body, or the *soma* in Shusterman's sense of the indivisible body–mind, all involve different systematised routines of aesthetic care for the body. These are often concerned with developing our sense of and sensitivity to our bodies, and include practices such as Buddhist meditation, yoga, the Feldenkrais method, and the Alexander technique. I do not intend to deal with these in detail here, but instead want to draw out one main concern with self-care and aesthetics.

If we take our own bodies as the main subject of our art, and our aesthetic experience is involved in caring for and shaping that body, we may be focused entirely introspectively on mental and physical states. This focus on ourselves and the attention to the health of our soma, is neither automatically a positive nor negative process. Any area of practice that extends from liposuction to Buddhist meditation is dealing with such diverse set of motivations and outcomes that it is important not to generalise too much about their common factors. A starting point here is, therefore, an acceptance that attention to one's own body is an aesthetic process and a vital means by which people engage aesthetically with their lives. It can become a resource for adjustment to the demands of the world, that is profoundly life enhancing. It can be a rigour that produces an enormous sense of contentment and joy, as well as being the source of terrible suffering and potential self-abuse. A discussion of self-care should not slip into an aesthetic appreciation that is based on standards of taste that might automatically disparage the practices of bodybuilder and endorse the skills of yoga practitioner. However, my point of departure is to suggest that in attempting to find a form of aesthetics that takes relationships seriously, the aesthetic fashioning of the self should not be the place from which we start. Shusterman certainly presents self-care as the leaping off point for a more sensitive relation to others. For him, 'creating individuals who are healthier and more flexibly open, perceptive, and effective through heightened somatic sensibility and mastery' (2000: 153) means they are more likely to be better citizens, more sensitive, or attuned to the needs of the world. It is, in his words, a short step from attention to 'one's own somatic efficacy' to 'effectively taking care of others' (2012: 190). While I expect there are instances when adequate or perhaps heightened attention to our own bodily welfare, through whatever means, might make someone more open and attentive to their place in wider society and the relations to others within it, my suggestion is that this should not be assumed. As I will mention below in a brief discussion of Japanese aesthetics, there might be a case to make from certain Japanese practices of self-care that this orientation to the other is an explicit expectation. However, self-care is just as likely to lead to forms of unsocial individualism, and even anti-social narcissism. In arguments for self-care being the first stage of a movement towards a greater openness to others, and a more selfless regard for their needs, the actual method for that leap from self to other is rarely explained sufficiently. This is taken up in discussion of what is called 'the gap' in Chapter 2. While I am not claiming empirical research that points to the contrary, I am sceptical of a suggestion that, put simply, is proposing that the more time someone spends in the gym, the more likely it is that he or she desires to build caring relations with others in their community. The move from the one to the other does not seem to have the guarantee suggested. So, for the aesthetics of care, care for the self is not a helpful starting point. Care aesthetics suggests a primary orientation to relations with others and moves on to discover what practices or routines might exist to enhance them. From attention to the aesthetics of these relations might come a focus on self-care as a necessary element, and not the other way around. The primary is relational, and the yoga, Alexander technique, and meditation disciplines are practices that might emerge, might be felt necessary extensions of, that basic condition of being *with* others. The importance of this will be developed in the following chapter in the discussion of care ethics and is discussed again below in relation to Japanese aesthetics, but here the emphasis is that care aesthetics is a search for the aesthetics of inter-human relations that does not take the aesthetics of creative self-fashioning as its starting point.

A return to objects

At the beginning of the chapter, I noted how the aesthetics in care aesthetics is primarily other focused rather than object focused. However, I also suggested that I did not want to dismiss aesthetics related to experience with objects entirely, and my opening examples of the axe and the potter hinted at this. While some object linked aesthetic theory does begin and end in our relation to those objects, there is also a considerable discussion of the way that attentiveness to the quality of the object can prompt a consideration of other people. Yuriko Saito's arguments for an everyday aesthetics suggest if we live amongst 'objects and environments expressive of care and thoughtfulness', we do not just contemplate those objects alone, but 'we tend to pass on kindness and consideration to those around us' (2017: 170). As with my argument about self-care above, the prompt for that tendency to pass on from object to person is rarely made as explicit at it could be. I am not doubting that it might happen but suggesting that in an account that sees an object's appreciation being linked to our sensitivity to others, it would be helpful for the mechanisms for this shift to be made clearer. When I witness the hands of Shoji Hamada manipulating clay, the proposition of Saito suggests that his gentle demeanour might also be evident in the quality of his relation to others. But again, there is a question as to how the quality of the care expressed in a gentle caress of the clay, becomes evidence of the quality of his relations with others or even the stimulus for a desire to develop a similar consideration in those relations. The contrary could also be the case. A person's ability to relate in a delicate and nurturing way with objects could be due to their lack of a similar capacity in interhuman relations.

One route to answering this question is to think through the role of the physiotherapist in my opening vignettes. In one sense, she was in relation to the object that was the hand of Antoine. Of course, the hand was of a person, and her careful massage of it was sustained through her precise touch, and intimate dealings with Antoine himself. If she had only dealt with it as a *mere* hand, a mere object, the suggestion is that the aesthetics of her care would have been diminished. It was her appreciation of it as an embodied hand, seeking reconnection to Antoine's missing fine motor skills, that ensured her precisely executed connection to it. In her massage there was a network of relations at play, between her and her own bodily capacity, specifically the skill in her hands, between her hand and Antoine's, and then between her wider sensory repertoire and Antoine's. The way the *object*, if we can call it that, was thus embedded in the broader relations between the two people, is perhaps a clue to how object relations may become part of the aesthetics of care as a relational, and interconnected human practice. Rather than thinking the hand as object, the demand here is to consider how we might think of objects more like hands, belonging to bodies, but also the connecting of the flesh between them.

One tradition in which this human–object–human relation is dealt explicitly is within the artistic and aesthetic practices of Japan. In selecting the aesthetics from one country for particular attention, the intention here is not to indicate that one tradition of aesthetics above many others is better placed to illustrate a version of aesthetics that resonates with the ambition of care aesthetics. An international analysis of various aesthetic traditions across multiple communities and cultures would be a worthy development from this proposal for care aesthetics and might be a challenge for future research. In many ways, the discussion above about the interaction of function and beauty, for example, is inspired by the different aesthetic approaches developed in indigenous scholarship (see Leuthold, 1998; Miner, 2017). A brief focus on Japan is, therefore, an illustration that different aesthetic traditions are vital for both testing and expanding the scope of this argument. Of course, any account of Japanese aesthetics such as this one is likely to fall into generalisations. There are both dangers of summative accounts as they tend to idealise aspects of aesthetic practices and also conceal others. In terms of Japan specifically, it is also important to be aware of the dangers of the projections of Japanese aesthetic practices beyond Japan, so well documented in the work of anthropologist Rupert Cox (2002). This is therefore admittedly an overbrief account and it will draw on a few texts that are close to the themes that have already been touched upon in this chapter. The purpose here is primarily to develop a space for an attention to objects in accounts of care aesthetics, which does not suffer from the limitations addressed earlier, and perspectives taken from certain commentaries on Japanese aesthetics are a helpful route to this. For those interested in a broader insight into Japanese aesthetics, the excellent readers edited by Nancy Hume (1995) and Michele Marra (1999), and historical contextual account from Eiko Ikegami (2005), are worthy starting points.

In the popular imagination, Japanese aesthetic practices range from martial arts such aikido and judo, to the tea ceremony and flower arranging, from visual arts as diverse as calligraphy and manga, and then to the performing arts such as Kabuki and Noh theatre. Some of these practices fall within the category we might call self-care discussed earlier, but even in these commentators such as Robert Carter (2007) and Shusterman (2012) maintain that the orientation developed through these disciplines leads to a certain sensitivity and care for the wider world. In some ways, my worry about the lack of inevitability in this move from personal discipline to social engagement might be countered by these Japanese examples where the physical disciplining of the self appears bound simultaneously to your relations with others. The flow of aikido between attack and response might be a case in point, but more broadly personal training in these *Zen arts* (Cox, 2002), whether focused on your own body or the craft of objects and environments, does propose that this enhances an attentiveness to one's place in the world. It is in the more intimate register of everyday aesthetics, however, that there appears to be a more fluid transference between careful attention to an object and the way this then confers your care to another. Carter in his account of *Japanese Arts and Self-Cultivation* concludes his study by announcing that Japan 'is still a culture that encourages a remarkable degree of other-directedness and caring' (1970: Loc. 1770). Whether this is empirically the case today, the point to take from this is that here we have an account of aesthetics that while it might start from care of the self, sees these relations as the route to more caring relations with others. Saito develops this through her writing on the small details of care for objects in the tea ceremony and more everyday behaviours such as 'opening and closing a door, holding a cup, serving a drink, giving and receiving a name card' (2017: 211). The sensory world of Japan, in her account, has multiple incidences of the embodied craft of interhuman relations. The object is thus not the single focused point of attention in these examples, and it is certainly not a distant, observed phenomena to provoke contemplation or appreciation. An object in Saito's version of aesthetics is, instead, felt, made, and *given*. The object is not on the wall, but passed between someone's fingers, through their hands and onto someone else. My concern expressed above about how inevitable the movement from self to other might be, is countered by an example where care for an object does not *infer* your care for another, but in fact *confers* your care onto them as it passes between you.

The notion of aesthetics located in how one's care for an object connects to an expression of the care you have for another is wonderfully documented in Joy Hendry's book *Wrapping Culture* (1993). She demonstrates the diverse cultures of wrapping within Japanese culture, from small souvenirs to major gifts for significant life events. While there are many different interpretations at play in this account, the act of wrapping can demonstrate your respect or affection for the person who receives the item, your desire to protect, and preserve the object itself, and also an attempt to ensure that unwrapping is a pleasant experience requiring its own care and dexterity. The object of a wrapped gift becomes the initiator of an aesthetic experience realised as an exchange of care – an *in between* experience to use the term from above. Instead of an account that is visually centric, the object itself becomes *wrapped* between people and part of the giving and taking, caring and receiving care, that flows across relationships. Of course, this process of reflecting closely on the impact of one's actions on the experiences of others suggests a certain culture of civility, or to use one of the terms in the subtitle of Hendry's book, *politeness*. Everyday practices of concern for the other in Japan, therefore, do not only become realised in a garden design's focus on the experience of the person walking through it, or the client in a tea ceremony enjoying the minute details of procedure tuned to their pleasure. It also results in micro moments of everyday action, rules of behaviour between people such as codes of etiquette, and linguistic practices of deference and respect. Saito links these patterns to a form of moral virtue so that the aesthetics of the everyday becomes an indicator of the quality of a 'good life' and a 'good society' (2008: 8). A concern I have here is that where certain behaviours are designated as moral virtues, there is a shift to a process of judgement that can easily become a disparagement of the sensory world of groups not deemed to have the correct aesthetic taste. As Saito is interested in how 'moral virtues such as respect, care, consideration, and thoughtfulness are often expressed, appreciated, and cultivated through *aesthetic means*' (2017: 150), we see a connection that while appropriately outlining the aesthetics of these daily behaviours, can too quickly impose the sensibilities of one, too often elite, group upon another. This is linked to the difference between a normative and a classificatory account of care aesthetics. The point to emphasise here is that in this account of concern for the other in daily acts of politeness and object sharing, we need to avoid establishing a regime of aesthetic judgement of these daily activities. We need to take care not to slip from a delight in the careful attention to the presentation of gifts, to a moral judgement of those that fail to meet the aesthetic standards of these modes of presentation.

The proposal for care aesthetics can be a normative account of 'good' care, or at minimum an appeal for a certain quality of care. By drawing on care ethics, as will be seen in the next chapter, the proposal must be dealing with some form of judgement because axiomatically it is challenging neat distinctions between the fields of ethics and aesthetics. However, the point to conclude with, is that the link between aesthetics and 'moral virtue' cannot rest in a transference where an aesthetic decision in one place neatly demonstrates virtue in a different register. Put simplistically, having perfectly polished shoes does not make you a good person. Similarly, giving a beautifully wrapped gift does not in and of itself becomes an indication of your virtue. If this were the case, seeing the shoes or the paper wrapping on the object would allow you to make a judgement of the wearer and the gift giver. Of course, people do this, and certainly do this far too much in terms of an aesthetics of everyday discrimination. Aesthetics here returns to the conceit of those trained with a delicacy of temperament enabling them to appreciate the true beauty of what they are seeing. It is again a reliance on the single distal sense of sight. Saito's 'respect, care, consideration, and thoughtfulness' cannot be a regime of propriety through which we judge others but instead must be considered as embodied experiences taking place between people. They can be aesthetically crafted, deeply sensory, and sensitive actions from one to another, a continuity between people, objects, and the world, but an assessment of their quality is dependent on those involved in the total experience and the sensory worlds in which they take place. What has been called 'negative aesthetics' (Berleant, 2011: Loc 2588) cannot be an attempt to reinstall an aesthetic judgement of taste via the backdoor of *politeness* in aesthetic experience of the everyday. The negative of experience can be acknowledged, but this must be through the account of those within the experience, and within the terms of the sensory affect and impact of the whole moment (and all the senses). The cleanliness of the nurse's attire does not determine and should not be read as a true signal of the sensory richness and quality of her professionalism. Sight alone, again, cannot be the only means to assess an understanding of aesthetic worth. Attention to her attire is but one sensory element of her whole demeanour. The aesthetic experience of care needs to take into account her full embodied engagement, including her affective disposition, her warmth, and responsiveness to a patient's desires. There is a complex and dynamic sensory repertoire which reaches across the moment to others at the point of care, and its virtue is not dependent on the witness to that moment. The *spectator* perceives one fraction of the aesthetic experience and ascertains *signs* of virtue which are as likely to be interpreted through the prism of their own prejudices and partial sensory norms. Notions of quality can only be located across and between all those engaged, and through attention to the expectations of the full sensory worlds that are at play. I absolutely want to argue that there can be a quality of aesthetic experience, and particular an experience of care which does nourish, support, and provide powerful, life-sustaining relations between people. And sensory experiences of this kind might expand capacities for more equitable lives or intervene where they are diminished. These are where aesthetic richness becomes a quality practice as understood and embodied by those participating in the moment. Collectively, this becomes a politics of a way of living that emerges in the unfolding of an aesthetic event.

One important point I did not mention in the analysis above, is that in suggesting that standards of *politeness* might introduce a problematic tone of moral indignation into this account, is that the Japanese for *polite* – *teinei* – can also be a synonym for care (Hendry, 1993: 64). So, however much I might seek some distance from the sensory world of etiquette and an account of care aesthetics, the overlap does need to be taken seriously. The Japanese world of politeness, in everyday actions and language, does have a connection to an embodied aesthetics of care and therefore where care prescribes social behaviours and might stratify what is considered worthy, commendable, or reproachable, the constraining power of care ethics and aesthetics should be noted. 'Be careful' is both an imperative that can enact unequal power relations as well as sustaining positive mutual concern. This of course is asking what it means to *take care*, and what is that care for others with which we are concerned. This is the subject of the chapter that follows.

To summarise this chapter, aesthetics in the pages that follow refers to a set of sensory experiences and perceptions that start with relations with people and not objects. Objects are still part of our focus but through the way that they confer relations between people and transfer care and affection across boundaries. Aesthetics in care aesthetics is about the total sensory world, and not just the arts, and is one where an aesthetic experience can take place in the smallest details of everyday life, or life changing, perhaps overwhelming events. These are bound into complex networks of social relations and do not occupy some realm apart from them. While an aesthetic experience can be heightened to the extent that it moves you beyond the moment you are in, this is not separate from the world, but dynamically in relation to it. An aesthetic experience engages all the senses, some more than others across the flow of the event and can seem to weave the functional with the beautiful in ways where one is difficult to untangle from the other. While care aesthetics is interested in self-care, it does not start from a fashioning of the individual body and move outwards to a subsequent care for the wider world. In being embedded in relations to others, it understands the aesthetics of self-care as potential development from the quality of our engagement with others. While the *aesthetics* of care aesthetics operates in an intimate register, so that the very slightest sensory acts of the everyday might be examples, it can also denote relations between groups and the sensory arrangements between people and the worlds in which they live. Aesthetics does not seek to delineate an appropriate style of behaviour or proscribe how people conduct themselves via codes of etiquette but hopes to find registers of kindness in daily lives that are meaningful for and shared by those involved each moment. The *aesthetics* of care aesthetics describes the sensory schema surrounding moments of care: small, momentary, or huge and systematic. Used in an honorific sense, as will be the predominate register in the pages that follow, it seeks to draw attention to sensory experiences that nourish, sustain, deepen, and enhance the quality of relations too often diminished in an aesthetically degraded world.

2

What is the *care* of care aesthetics?

In the opening section of the previous chapter, I offered several examples that illustrated moments when care and aesthetics were brought together and where a practice could be assessed as having both a care component and an aesthetics. This required a certain interpretation of the aesthetic realm and what it meant to designate an experience *aesthetic*. Only by outlining a particular view of aesthetics could my case for an aesthetics of care be made. This chapter has a comparable purpose. It seeks to outline a particular vision of care, primarily drawn from the field of care ethics, to make the case that care can be legitimately considered for its aesthetics. Like that word, care is beset by histories of usage, assumptions of meaning, and dangers of both lack of clarity and perhaps overfamiliarity. The purpose of this chapter is to outline a version of care that is both important for understanding of contemporary society, but also one that sustains and is hopefully enhanced through an understanding of its aesthetic dimensions. A difference between the two chapters of Part 1 is that in writing of aesthetics, there was a particular and at times non-mainstream reading of aesthetic theory adopted. It was written against certain versions of aesthetic theory to make a case that care could be understood aesthetically. The direction here is somewhat different in that I am writing *with the grain* of care ethics, accepting many of its propositions, but then offering elements of additional focus, particularly around notions of embodiment, that themselves come from within this philosophical discipline. For those familiar with the care ethics field, there will be some well-trodden ground in the pages that follow, but I hope there is sufficient new emphasis that will be of interest.

Care is used in so many different formulations and is such a commonplace term that trying to draw a boundary around it to fix its meaning is daunting and, in some ways, a futile task. Barely will a day go by without it being heard in a diversity of somewhat disconnected contexts. It is used in endless expressions,

DOI: 10.4324/9781003260066-4

colloquialisms, and teenage shoulder shrugs: think 'who cares', 'why should I care', and 'I couldn't care less'. It is the anodyne title of numerous social policy practices from 'care in the community' and 'care homes', to 'kids in care' and 'care packages'. It is part of our everyday life as we care for our children or worry about elder care. We might act as informal carers, be paid as carers for others, seek carers for our loved ones, or need personal care ourselves. It is the sight of controversy as carers abuse their charges and vice versa as care workers are exploited as migrant labour, with limited rights often far from their homelands. Its ubiquity hints at its importance, but also invisibility. It contains a demand – we should care for this or for that – but it is also decried as a burden as we hope to forget our cares or to become more carefree. It is the nexus of deep inequality as insisting one person cares for another, or one category of people care for another, suggest hierarchies of power and control which may discriminate against both carers and the cared-for. The focus on care reminds us of a history of feminist scholarship that was both identifying the private realm as worthy of attention and noting those activities largely done by women as demanding more systematic analysis. As will be discussed below the care ethics field is indebted to this history of scholarship and activism. Similarly, care has become a rallying cry for political change as we are petitioned to care for the future of the planet or distribute care more equitably so that *black lives matter*. It is an economic transaction as we pay carers, and it is an unpaid commitment to care for loved ones. While it can be a call to action, to care about injustice, it is also an excuse for inaction as we might care, but simultaneously believe that nothing can actually be done. It is used normatively – suggesting something worthy or intrinsically positive, but it is also used purely descriptively. Care might designate an act with no automatic insight as to whether it was done well or poorly. A person might be *caring* for an elder but do so without any sense of their dignity or even consent. Alternatively, they might do it with great skill and attention to the complex needs and aspirations of the individual.

To work through this web of different usages and problematic implications, the chapter will outline the history of the field called care ethics that has grown up around a group of feminist scholars since the 1980s. This is not to assert that there is a fixed consensus about the meaning and importance of care for contemporary society amongst this very diverse group of writers, but to draw up certain parameters for how care might be understood as part of the complexity of our lives, and in turn how it might be understood aesthetically. This will include the development of different definitions of care ethics, and how they have changed over time. The chapter will outline how care ethics came to be linked to certain gendered notions of behaviour and identity, and then how it moved away from the association of care with any 'natural' capacity of women. For an account that is looking at care as creating aesthetic experience, it needs to reject the proposition that it is solely a capacity of certain groups. The chapter will discuss the implications of care as a practice, linked to the care of the self (of course referring to the aesthetics of self-fashioning in the previous chapter), as well as objects and human others. It will outline care's relationality and how it proposes a form of interdependence that stands against assumptions of autonomy as the idealised purpose of human life. This parallels the discussion of aesthetics as heteronomous and *in between* in the previous chapter. While understanding care requires an analysis of how it materialises in intimate practices between individuals, and this will certainly be important for the case for care aesthetics, care will also be described as a network of social practices which have significance for the organisation of communities and wider society. The chapter will conclude with an exploration of how care as a practice needs to understand the role of the body more explicitly, to attend to the affective components of care, and thus how care can be performed or be understood for its aesthetic qualities. There are multiple instances in the care literature of care being discussed in aesthetic terms and these will be outlined, but importantly there are accounts from the care ethics literature where the aesthetic nature of care is either denied or disparaged. This chapter will, inevitably, argue against the suspicion of care as *mere performance* or a somewhat commonplace idea of the aesthetic of care as antithetical to an ethic of care. The chapter ends with a turn from caring between people, to how we might care for our world and whether these are complementary or opposed. This will lead to a proposal for a politics of care ethics that is making a particular critique of tendencies in contemporary society and how a politically attuned understanding of care aesthetics is necessary. The ambition is that the account here combined with previous chapter will establish an overview of care aesthetics that while not complete, provides a firm enough touchstone for the analysis in the following chapters focusing on the arts, health and social care, and the everyday.

In suggesting briefly both the ubiquity of its use and diversity of contexts in which the concept of care is found, one of the first perspectives on care ethics is illustrated. A primary claim is that care is, in the words of Judith Philips, 'part of everyone's life' (2007: 169). Care is not a peculiar or parochial concern of certain groups, but a common experience of all humankind. All experience the care of a parent, biological, or otherwise, and while for some it will be powerfully nurturing, warm, and life sustaining, and for others it will be beset by neglect, cursory attention, and at worse abuse, the human animal is unique in the time and intensity of support which is necessary for us to reach adulthood. A common experience of care, whatever its quality, is followed by further care experiences as many will need care during adult life, and most will require additional forms of care if lucky enough to survive into old age. The critical input of care ethicists is to assert that care is unremarked because it is hidden in the private sphere and therefore denied public import, and secondly that it can be the source of context-dependent ethics that work against the universalist claims of traditional ethical theories. Care, according to these theories, should not be an invisible backdrop to a successful appearance in a world of public action and behaviour, but the critically examined and commented upon enabling factor that sustains us through different stages of our lives. Who does it, how it is done, who needs it, who provides it, and what happens when it is either present or absent, demands attention and critical enquiry. One purpose of *Care Aesthetics* is to insist that while the attention to care is somewhat obvious in the health and social care field, this *who*, *how*, and *what* of care should also be considered within the socially engaged arts.

Two of the earliest proponents of an ethics of care, Nell Noddings and Carol Gilligan, who came from backgrounds in education and psychology respectively, have been credited with setting out many of the parameters for an approach to ethics that challenged assumptions about how ethical behaviour might be understood. Gilligan in her pioneering work on women's moral reasoning, challenged both the exclusion of women and girls from standard portrayals of the development of young people's responses to moral dilemmas (exemplified in her collaboration with the psychologist of moral development, Lawrence Kolberg) and the idea that their tendency to see 'a world comprised of relationships rather than of people standing alone, a world that coheres through human connection rather than through systems of rules' (2009: 29) was somehow inferior. While the extent that this propensity is part of a natural or innate women's voice can be questioned, her case studies and work with young women should be valued as a counter to what she called the 'repeated exclusion of women from the critical theory-building studies of psychological research' (Ibid: 1). Here we have an echo of Irigaray from Chapter 1, where pointing out that theory building that has excluded women does not make a claim for an essentialist women's capacity but indicates the partialness of one that only relies on perspectives derived from studies dominated by men.

Nel Noddings' work similarly explored the different moral registers that become apparent when one focuses on the attributes and behaviours traditionally associated with women. Her pioneering work on caring, which in the 1984 edition of her book was called a 'feminine approach to ethics and moral education', started from an analysis of the moral capacities that are revealed if we focus on a simple dyad of what she labelled the 'one-caring' and the 'cared-for' (2013: 4). She argued that 'a powerful and coherent ethic and, indeed, a different sort of world may be built on the natural caring so familiar to women' (Ibid: 46) and while we may reject caring as *natural*, we need to extract the insight that activities of care (familiar to women but not necessarily chosen or innate) can lead to insights about how humans might relate, support, and draw strength from each other. While Noddings renamed future editions of her book 'a relational approach to ethics' to counter accusations of gender essentialism, we need to credit both her and Gilligan for demonstrating that a realm in which women were traditionally restricted could be the source of ethics. This was not to say that women should be happy with caring roles for the unique insight into morality that it might give them, but that the knowledge of people who do care could be a resource for understanding how people might learn to relate and sustain each other. In fact, the ambition explicit in the quotation above is far from parochial as it asserts that care ethics aims to build a *different kind of world*. In starting from this point, care ethics offered a new way of valuing context, situatedness, and relationally dependent behaviours that were dismissed as irrelevant by traditional ethics. A sensitivity to context countered a system of universally agreed rules that were to be rationally applied by individuals unfettered by concerns for others. These early works can be critiqued for a tendency to view women's roles, as mothers for example, as a fixed, natural state. However, the insight that propelled future care ethics work was set by an assertion that caring behaviours, whether parental, occupational, or voluntary, while unequally distributed and unfairly resourced, might provide inspiration for how more equitable ethical, inter-human relations could be developed.

Care ethics moved on from these early writers to question the place of both gender and what was seen to be the narrow focus on a dyadic relationship between two people. While the feminist origins of care ethics should not be overlooked, writers like Selma Sevenhuijsen argued for 'uncoupling care from symbolic forms of femininity, and at the same time listening to women's multiple voices in social practices of caring' (2003: 19). She aimed to place care in terms of citizenship (Ibid: 15) and similarly one of the key writers on care ethics, Jean Tronto, sought to question how care can be taken away from the home (2013: 6). While expanding an understanding of care beyond archetypes of 'mother/child' and similar gendered roles, so that care ethics might deal with care in multiple settings across numerous different forms of relation, we should not dismiss the relation of parent to child or the caring that does happen in the home, but instead include these practices within the multiple, interrelated contexts in which care does take place. Women still in many settings, whether formal or informal, domestic or public, do make a disproportionate contribution to care and that is a problem to be addressed and set of practices to be explored. Peta Bowdens' work on 'gender sensitive ethics' acutely demonstrates this by showing the different ways that care is played out in different relational contexts. Rather than a single ethic of care, she illustrates 'the ethical irreducibility of specific situations' (2008: 3) and through analyses of actual practices in mothering, friendship, nursing, and citizenship, she demonstrates the different forms of care and different ethical questions that each give rise to, without naturalising women's roles in their execution (Ibid: 12). For an account that seeks to demonstrate an aesthetic of these care practices, it is vital that this plural and situation-sensitive approach to care ethics is acknowledged.

Writers such as Virginia Held and Fiona Robinson have sought to draw care ethics into broader social relations, so that concerns for the field might include 'medical practice, law, political life, the organization of society, war, and international relations' (Held, 2006: 9) where 'the transformatory potential of an ethics of care extends beyond the personal to the political and, ultimately, to the global context of social life' (Robinson, 1999: 23). In my desire to connect care ethics to the community-based practice of artists and health care workers, this shift is significant but also it is important to note that many of the primary definitions still rely on formulations that appear to endorse a somewhat singular dyadic caring relation. In Noddings' work, this can be found in the idea of the one-caring and the cared-for, and her difficulty in ascribing an ethic to the activity of 'caring about' (2013: 141) because this implied a relation with distant others for whom one would struggle to create any form of 'person-to-person contact' (Ibid). Proximal, person-to-person connection, was, therefore, central to her definition of care. Similarly, Tronto's early categories of care which included caring about, caring for, caregiving, and care receiving (2013: 21), all appear to be interpersonal rather than communal or social. She does add 'caring with' (Ibid: 23) suggesting the importance of meeting care needs at a broader societal level, but this reads as an addition to her original schema rather than a core feature of care practice. The tension between care discussed in an intimate personal relationship register and approaches that demand a more social or collaborative practice will be an important recurring theme in the discussion below. The challenge is to view care as personal and yet multiple simultaneously, in a form of what Eva Kittay has called 'nested' practices (2015: 52). Care is exercised in ways that are embedded within and connected to each other, so even expanding care's purview to include the *organisation of society or international relations* must acknowledge the multiple proximal relations nested within it. For care aesthetics, this is important as it seeks to value intimate practices of care alongside the group based, institutional and social.

In Jean Tronto's four (and later five) elements of care, first outlined in her book *Moral Boundaries*, she suggests that each aspect of care needs an 'ethical element' (1993: 127) for it to be effective. To 'care about' with any degree of success, people need the quality of *attentiveness* which is where one recognises 'in the first place that care is necessary' (Ibid: 106). Then, to care for someone, one needs to assume 'responsibility for the identified need' (Ibid) and be willing to determine how one might respond to it. Then, to give care one needs the capacity to meet the actual needs for care, which includes a set of appropriate skills, so Tronto outlines, by way of example, 'the nurse administering medication, the repair person fixing the broken thing, the mother talking to her child about the day's events, the neighbour helping a friend to set her hair' (Ibid: 107). Finally, to receive care one needs a quality of responsiveness, so that you are in a position to respond to the care given in a way that ensures one has a particular need met. These care capacities can be understood in light of Tronto's widely quoted definition of care that she developed with her colleague Berenice Fisher:

> we suggest that caring be viewed as a *species activity that includes everything we do to maintain, continue, and repair our 'world' so that we can live in it as well as possible.* That world includes out bodies, our selves, and our environment, all of which we seek to interweave in a complex, life-sustaining web
>
> *(1993: 103. Italics in the original).*

The point to emphasise here is that however broadly focused her definition (up to and including everything done to repair the world), ultimately many of the practices she outlines, and the space for ethical behaviour she describes, relies on an attentive person responsive or competent to meet the care needs of others. The question is how we might allow the definitions that seem to apply to dyadic relations, one person to another, that are crucial for some examples of care, to work for nested caring relations between and among multiple people. Tronto's definition is important for an argument for care aesthetics because it starts to hint that the skills required for a practice of care have a sense of craft. Being competent, attentive, and responsive might be descriptors of the artist as they engage their materials or their participants. They certainly were features of the vignettes that introduced the previous chapter. Similarly, the *maintaining, continuing and repairing of the world* can be understood to require a certain set of embodied skills that can shape and mend – again a suggestion of a craft-like capacity. The challenge, something to be developed below, is how attentiveness of another, what Noddings refers to as 'engrossment' (2013: 12), might translate to the interactions at a level beyond the inter-personal. Later why the focus only on care between two people might be a problem is explained for the broader ambition of both care ethics and care aesthetics, but there is another question raised by this focus that needs to be addressed first.

The second challenge posed by the Tronto and Fischer definition is that in focusing on the capacities of the one caring, and how they respond and attend, and what care does to the world, it maintains a focus on the carer as central or primary. They are able to make judgements 'about needs, conflicting needs, strategies for achieving ends' (1993: 137) in a way that suggests that they have the power, the agency, to do so. While it is important to note in the carer-cared for dyad that the hierarchy between the one in need and the one who meets those needs, is a site of potential inequality and at worst abuse, Tronto is right in her account to show how we need to question where the inequality lies in this relationship. She pointedly demonstrates that carers are frequently poorly paid women, migrant workers, and people of colour who are liable to be vulnerable to the economic power of those for whom they care. As she states bluntly, 'those who are least well off in society are disproportionately those who do the work of caring' and then on the other side of this relationship 'the best off members of society often use their positions of superiority to pass caring work off to others' (Ibid: 113). So, the dyad in her work is in fact one where any assumed hierarchy between carer and cared-for, needs to be parsed with attention to the dynamics of both economics and class, gender, and race. I make this point because a definition of care that speaks of competencies and attentiveness, and then responsiveness on the part of the care receiver, fails if it does not consider that many who live in these relationships do not do so through a free desire to attend, but through the exigencies of a global economy that demands some are paid to administer the care for others. We need to understand that 'making judgments' (Ibid: 137) makes a demand on carers without noticing that they might not have the freedom to make those judgements, or the terms of that judgement are made for them, as this was not a relationship into which they entered freely. We may ask, how might they enact a caring relation, and how might the care receiver respond, in spite of the complex lines of control that determine the type of care that is practiced. Care ethics, and subsequently care aesthetics, while usefully focusing on capacity and competencies of care, must examine how these are played out through dynamics of power and inequality. If we solely focus on the attentiveness of the carer for her or his charge as a central definition of that relation, we remain fixed with a free choice version of care, linked primarily to voluntaristic models, such as those between the parent and child. While voluntary relations might be common examples through which care ethics can demonstrate its situated morality, they cannot be the sole archetype. This problem of the dyad and the sole focus on the carer is taken up again in Chapter 4 in the discussion of the 'art of the nurse'.

Care and justice

In staking out the ground for an ethics of care, proponents compared it to an alternative, which was, in Gilligan's words, 'an ethics of rights' (2009: 164). Care ethics was set against a justice model of ethics, where the latter revolved around a competition of interests between freely interacting individuals. Gilligan's work on the voice of women proposed 'two different moral ideologies' (Ibid) so that a situated, context-dependent, and relational approach to moral decision-making was a counter to generalisable, individualistic, and rule-based ethics located in fixable notions of what was just. Virginia Held summed up this division as follows:

> whereas an ethic of justice seeks a fair solution between competing individual interests and rights, an ethic of care sees the interests of carers and cared-for as importantly intertwined rather than as simply competing. Whereas justice protects equality and freedom, care fosters social bonds and cooperation
>
> *(2006: 15).*

In seeking to position care as a new site of moral deliberation and action, there was a danger in these accounts that they could be read as suggesting that care ethics somehow rejected a commitment to justice. However, by pointing out the importance of an awareness of the inequalities that can exist in caring relations above, the aim is to insist that care ethics is not opposed to justice ethics. In fact, a commitment to just relations should be taken to the heart of the demand that more caring communities need to be built. Rather than position care ethics dichotomously against justice ethics, it is the assumptions drawn for a traditional approach to justice that needs to be challenged. As Fiona Robinson writes, 'it is not the idea of "justice" as such' which care ethics is opposed to, but rather 'the individualist, atomistic ontology, the liberal-impartial view of persons as "generalized" rather than "concrete", and the concomitant reliance on abstract moral principles which are corrected by the care perspective' (1999: 25).

Care ethics stays with the particular and is not afraid of it as the site of competing, complex, and dynamically shifting ethical practices and deliberations. This does not make it narrow, but rather an ethics linked to how people live their lives with and between each other in ways that are geographically, historically, and culturally situated.

Care as practice

In the opening account of the different uses of the word care, it was noted that caring for something did not automatically mean that one would do something about it. To care was not synonymous with to act. This is the disjuncture described in Noddings' work as the difference between caring about, which she would argue might not include any activity, and caring for, which involves a specific set of actions. To make a case for care having an aesthetics, the insistence here will be that there is an activity or practice of care, which cannot be neatly extracted from the values that promote care, or the affective experience of it. In fact, the desire to care does not automatically precede a caring act but might be concurrent with it, or post-act product of it. Following Held, care needs to be understood as both a 'cluster of practices' and a 'cluster of values' (2006: 4) that are imbricated across moments of activity. Rather than understanding 'caring about' as flawed because it fails as an act, the position here is to see expressions of care, spoken, written, and proposed, as not discontinuous from physical activities and possible affective responses that might emerge from an experience of care. Care does not neatly fall into a linear human endeavour of decision-based agency, where we desire or are called to care, where we then enact that care and subsequently reflect or respond to it. The economies, inequalities, physicality, and cultural norms that are woven through examples of care cannot be reduced to neat voluntaristic human controlled timelines moving from desire, to act and to result. Care is an activity but not a 'set of principles which can simply be followed' (Sevenhuijsen, 2003: 107) and while we might aspire, for example, for it to be an 'important practice of contemporary citizenship' (Robinson, 1999: 81) we cannot preordain how care as a complex experiential process will unfold. Care will be, therefore, considered a practice in these pages in much the same way that my focus on aesthetics concentrated on experience. It is a doing and a done-to reaching between and beyond individuals as they simultaneously prepare, repair, and remake relationships within families, communities, and wider society. It can be done by the care assistant bathing an older person and it can be experienced by the youth in a theatre group as they work together on a performance.

One aspect of care that was commented upon extensively in the previous chapter was the notion of self-care, or the *fashioning of the self*. This was connected to the movement of somaesthetics and the idea of one's own body, and life, as a work of art, and draws indirectly on Foucault's work in Volume 3 of his history of sexuality called '*The Care for the Self*' (1990). The argument in

Chapter 1 doubted whether aesthetic self-fashioning could be the preliminary work that might enable people to engage more fully with or orientate themselves to the world. Ella Myers, in her work on what she calls 'worldly ethics', refers to a position within care ethics that grants 'chronological primacy to ethical self-intervention' (2013: 44) as 'therapeutic ethics' (Ibid: 48) and affirms this critique. She argues that a form of care politics that starts with the self cannot be a starting point for a project of care for the world, where this orientation might lead to what for her would be progressive forms of democratic association. She is hinting at a problem that is present across the care literature, which is how care within one setting might relate to care in another. If you care for your children, does this make you more likely to care for the children of others? If you receive care from a friend, does this make you more likely to practice care for another? If you are practiced at intimate care, does this open you to care for the planet? If you care for yourself, does this prepare you for care for distant or even immediate others? Myers' book is an account of the persistent failure of this movement, where one's capacity for self-care or interpersonal care makes no automatic transformation into an ability or interest in caring for society, or in her terms, 'care for the world' (Ibid: 85). Here I want to both accept aspects of her argument but also push back at its pessimism. While it might be hard to demonstrate that one's skills at intimate care, say, of a grandparent ensures that you might exhibit a capacity to care for other elders, the case for care aesthetics seeks to demonstrate that there is a connection between the intimate and the more social.

Some writers support the idea of a flow from one practice of care to the others. So, for example, Graham Longford in his work on cruel aesthetics, exploring Foucault's work in particular, argues that self-care helps 'dislodge us from our habitual centers of gravity' (2001: 589) which in turn enables a realisation that all identities are contingent. However, the mechanism that moves a person from a focus on their identity to an understanding of others, or from self-care to openness to the care for needs of others, is not made explicit. The position here, as discussed in Chapter 1, is that there can be nothing given about this shift. Myers is right in her assertion that 'the connection between self-care and socio-political dynamics is only weakly and inconsistently articulated'. (2013: 23) and we are wrong to assume that 'the turn inward will give way to a turn outward' (Ibid: 43). This is not only a problem of self-care, but also as mentioned above, aspects of micro or proximal care and how they might shift into concern for broader social realms. Tronto repeats the confidence of Longford when she asserts that experience of giving or receiving care makes us both more skilled at caring and also 'more caring and moral people' and 'better citizens in a democracy' (1993: 167). How one morphs to the other, how we turn the intimate register dial to meet this concern with democratic politics is one of the challenges of the case for care aesthetics. How do crafted, artful relations between people at the level of interpersonal intimacy, metamorphose into proclivities to wider social concern or a desire to *repair*, or even change, the world? While this movement is assumed more than explained, the position here is to question the pessimism of an account that it is unlikely or even impossible. The ambition of care aesthetics is that it does connect the interpersonal and intimate with broader practices of care across communities.

In discussing self-care, the argument is that there is no inherent connection between looking after oneself and a concern to care for others or the wider world. Yoga class attendance, gym memberships, and pre-occupation with personal grooming might prepare a person for an orientation to issues of the wider world or enhance a capacity to engage more socially, but they are also the premium activities of a society that values atomistic individualism. As stated in Chapter 1, they are as likely to produce narcissistic introspection as an openness to others. While the perspective here is not to dismiss self-care, the emphasis is on care as an ethic where our relation to others is its primary feature. Rather than one drawn from the challenges faced by an autonomous agent standing alone, even when focused on a care for themselves, it insists that one's relations to others are ontologically given. We are born into a world, and survive in that world, in relation to the people and the features of the context in which we a located. Sevenhuijsen sets this in broader terms where the 'stable, complete and unlimited self of universal ethics' is replaced by a different vision, by a 'multiple and ambiguous moral self, who is aware of his or her own limitations, dependencies, vulnerability and finiteness' (2003: 57). The starting point for an argument that suggests that a movement between capacities of intimate interpersonal care and wider care for groups, communities and society is possible, is this insistence that 'care is a relational ethic' (Hamington, 2014: 198) and that in the words of Gilligan, we understand the world as 'comprised of relationships rather than of people standing alone' (2009: 29). To progress this argument, the next section will start from the micro implications of this relational ontology by discussing intimate relations and the importance of tactile knowledge. It will then move onto care as networked practices and extend this to explore caring solidarity. This will lead to a discussion of the importance of the notion of interdependence where care ethics posits the inevitable dependencies that shape human and non-human relations against a vision of autonomy and independence. The shift from the intimate to the broader social networked vision of care is not presented as a continuum, but as an outline of a continuity. Care operates as a finely woven mesh of practices where matters of scale should not be assumed to imply significance or priority. Unlike Myers who insists on 'world care' as the chronologically prior, and therefore motivating and binding activity of other 'lesser' care practices, the argument here is that care cannot be unpicked in this way. Inevitably, this meshed approach to a care ecosystem provides the terrain into which my approach to care aesthetics must find its place.

Intimate care

Care is frequently discussed in an intimate register where we act to support and nurture those close to us (both familiarly and professionally). Intimacy in this sense can be a physically proximal relation to a person, but one can also exhibit intimacy with object, as a curator might with the items in her care or as a potter like Shoji Hamada did with his clay. It might also be intimacy with ideas as a writer might feel as they craft prose or poetry, or with geographies as people might sense an intimate and embedded relation to a neighbourhood or wider environment. Intimacy, however, is most often understood as an embodied quality of a physical relationship. The way people are intimate with each other can demonstrate a range of qualities of attention and concern, and this is important for the aesthetics of care because it is through intimate relations that there can be a certain crafted focus on the shape of an experience. In terms of care ethics, a focus on intimacy is a challenge to the assumption that ethics only happens in public between free autonomous individuals. Here, close relations of care become a site through which ethics is enacted and demonstrated and at their best these include attention, respect, concern for others, and responsiveness. Of course, an account of intimacy must not deny how there are opportunities for this relation to be one of inequality, abuse, fear, and one where concern might be a mask for control or coercion. Attention to intimacy must reveal these multiple possibilities rather than assuming it as an automatic good. Similarly, in pointing out the importance of the intimate encounter for the case for care aesthetics and noting this can be an 'artful' practice, I am claiming this as an important but not the only mode through which care aesthetic experiences are realised. Intimacy is one register through which caring behaviours are enacted.

When discussing intimacy, it is important not to assume that it is a *natural* capacity and to caution against a view that it is the particular propensity of certain groups or individuals. For example, while the parent–child relation may be an experience of intimacy, it is not automatically so. Similarly, a mother or father are not pre-ordained to effect intimate care, simply due their biological relations to a child. To avoid this assumption of inherent capacity, Julia Twigg uses the expression *bodywork* to define practices of intimate care done by care workers as part of what, with her collaborator Christina Buse, she labels the 'close tactility' of care (2018: 341). Their analysis focused on paid intimate care work, an important reminder that intimate relations might be voluntary, paid, between family members or between strangers. Care ethics seeks to analyse the experience of intimacy and elicit the values and attributes that are exercised through it. This might be parent to child, but it might also be poorly paid care worker to wealthy elder employer. By focusing here on its tactile nature, attention is drawn to how the body at work in these relations is so often overlooked. As Hamington notes, 'the subtleties needed to offer a caring hug, look, touch, or comportment of the body are largely unarticulated' (2015: 54) and while it is unremarkable to note that much 'caring involves both physical touch and bodily tending' (Barnes, 2015: 38), the shape, feel, and quality of that tending are missed from much analysis. The claim here is that the bodywork of intimate attention to the needs of another rarely focuses sufficiently on the affective and sensory components of that practice. To understand its successes and failures, qualities and challenges, these *aesthetic* elements of the encounter need to be better understood.

Accounts of the practice of intimate care range from Hamington's familial 'hug' (2004: 57) to Twigg's analysis of the close work of 'bathing, washing and other forms of person care' (2000: 394). These intimacies dealt with in further detail in Chapter 4, whether with a loved relative, a paying client, or a vulnerable patient often involve some form of touching. While this section will briefly focus on the significance of that touch for care ethics and aesthetics, a focus on this connection, again, notes that it can be an unwanted physical breech as much as a soothing caress. The act of touching and being touched is important for an ethic of care and may be pleasurable or unpleasurable. It is a productive, complex, and occasionally fraught site of interpersonal connection, realised in what María Puig de la Bellacasa argues is a form of intimate knowledge making. She defines touch as 'a sense of material-embodied relationality' that 'eschews abstractions and detachments that have been associated with dominant epistemologies of knowledge-as-vision' (2017: 390). The claim to make is not that touch is a form of primary knowledge practice, or a foundational aspect of human relations, but that it is an overlooked practice that has its own dynamics, capacities, and formal aspects, which are vital for the focus on the aesthetics of care. This edition, when dealing with touch, acknowledges it has an extensive literature, from the psychological and philosophical to the technical and practical. As *Care Aesthetics* is both a theoretical proposition and an account of practice, it draws on different traditions, but primarily orientates to the sociologies of touch from writers in the field of social care (see Twigg, 2002; Twigg et al, 2011). In terms of care ethics, an attention to touch focuses on an encounter where the 'distinctions between "I" and "You"' become blurred (Harari, 2011: 142), so that it is inevitably an inter-relational practice. This emphasis explains why, following the previous chapter and the comments earlier, the experience of care is the unit of analysis rather than the capacities of an individual carer. Touch reminds us that care is created by the carer and the cared-for, and sole focus on the capacity of one misses this inter-relation. Chapter 4 develops this approach when discussing the problematic concept of the art of the nurse and how it links to bodywork. The insistence here that touch is never straightforwardly from one to another, indicates why care aesthetics is more interested in how the carer and the cared-for co-create the caring moment. In more practically orientated literature in this area, there is a greater sense of what the touch of one person offers another, for example as a means for meeting people's 'emotional and physical needs' (Tanner, 2017: 127) where they can be diminished by a culture where touch is restricted or prohibited. However, touch here will pivot between these different approaches, focusing both on how health and social care writers have explored touch as a care practice and acknowledging that it has the intersubjective characteristics, linked to the blurring of the categories of 'I' and 'you' developed by writers such as Harari.

Where touch decentres our sense of self, care ethics seeks a similar decentring away from the singular, rational individual capable of making correct judgement. This is an argument for a more fully embodied understanding of ethical relations. As Hamington notes, 'we use our voice, posture, hands, and arms, as well as our minds in order to care' (2012: 34) and each of these is entwined within a complex moment of practice. While this might be enacted spontaneously within a flow of encounter between people, in what Pink and colleagues have called 'tactile knowing' (2014: 438), care ethics proposes that this is central to ethical inquiry. These moments are not mere private matters of insignificant personal concern, but crucial human endeavours which practice and exhibit a series of ethical exchanges. While there may be externally formulated rules or norms of behaviour that govern each moment, particularly if the practice occurs in a professional setting, these in fact rarely script simplistically from learnt–rule to embodied action. Instead, the particularity of any given context demands certain practices of touching and embodied care, governed by multiple peculiarities of skill, experience, timing, prior relations, and situated knowledge, that in turn generate and demonstrate the ethical dynamics of the moment. As tactile knowledge is always experienced between people, between people and objects and then wider environments (see Sedgwick, 2003), it may include aspects of equality, reciprocity, and responsiveness and, of course, may enact more problematic and damaging behaviours. In making the claim that the work of touch operates in these ways, and can contribute to the 'affective, symbolic and communicatory work of health care' (Pink, Morgan and Dainty, 2014: 431), the proposal for care aesthetics asks the follow up question of *how* these moments are made possible and by what skills and capacities they might be sustained. *Tactile knowing* is a co–created experience made by different individuals across multiple contexts, and care aesthetics wants to know *how* that knowing is practiced, what forms it takes in different moments, and what pressures it faces in different social or political settings. It claims touch in contexts of care might be a responsively crafted, with different levels of precision or finesse, and these are insufficiently noted and valued. By drawing them to our attention and analysis, they might then be acknowledged as more crucial elements of the ethical relations that the experiences of care might enact. These debates will be returned to in Chapter 4 in the discussion of care aesthetics in contexts of health and social care.

In Noddings' work on care ethics, she uses a slightly different understanding of touch and this is useful in demonstrating a link between actual physical touch, and the idea of being more metaphorically *in touch* with an event or person. She argues in a chapter titled *what does it mean to care,* that to care is 'to be touched, to have aroused in me something that will disturb my own ethical reality' (2013: 14). She suggests an affective call to care that challenges the boundaries of the self, and disturbs an ethical reality solely situated within one's own body. While attention to another can elicit this response, it should not be taken to imply that this level of physically aroused concern is inevitable or innate to any particular type of person. Similarly, it is not to forget that care might be an economic exchange where any sense of affective call might be imbricated with contracts, formal regulations and hourly wages that can make sensed, spontaneously felt concern difficult to discern. However, the point to make here is that touch as physical hand-on-body work and the feeling of being in touch with someone, even at a distance, are interwoven aspects of care relations and part of the complexity of the way that care is networked between people and the communities in which they live. Touch is therefore not to be understood as literal *or* metaphorical but a continuity of practices which might include the skill of hands – the physiotherapist or the masseur – and felt connections across intimate relations and wider networks of association. The sensation of connection is not only to be associated with proximal relations with a single individual. Understanding care as a network is important because it extends care relations beyond a purely dyadic, person to person, version of care practices, to insist that care is also realised between interconnected people and is woven into the caring that expands across the contexts in which they live. These networks are not necessarily an even web of relations, bonded between different people in equally, mutually reinforcing patterns. They are more often distributed unequally across both time and space, so that one person might give care to multiple others far more frequently than their peers, or some may need more care at different moments, and some may be forced to migrate to provide care, leaving family members in the care of others. Care is a complex network and analysing it reveals inequalities which are differentially distributed between nations, groups, and communities. We need that network to survive, because as Judith Butler writes 'our persistence as living organisms depends on the matrix of sustaining interdependent relations' (2015: 86) and that means we should seek to strengthen its touchpoints and interconnections in such a way as to respond to or counter the inequalities that woven through it. Those nodes might be exhibited in the craft of physical touch or experienced through the affective response of *being in touch* or completing actions that *touch the lives* of multiple others.

Suggesting that care should be understood as a network of relations is not to dismiss the dyadic relationship – between say teacher and student or nurse and patient. The approach here is that the dyad is important part of the practice of caring relations, a vital part of its aesthetics, and it is simultaneously an element within that wider network. One might benefit from the care given to your own children that enables you to go to work, while also shopping for an infirm neighbour and being part of a group that meets to develop mutual care for each other in relation to a particular experience or history. There are multiple relations between different groups of people at play at any one time, and the aesthetics of those relations take different shapes, and structure different experiences. They are part of what the previous chapter called a sensory world. Myers approach is different in that she disregards the dyadic relation as a contributing relation to an ethic of care. She locates the focus on one-to-one care in the work of Emmanuel Levinas and criticises it as a form of charitable ethics; one that relies on the 'asymmetrical relation of obligation to a unique Other' (2013: 64). This is a restatement of the argument from earlier in the chapter, which suggested that if the care remained tied purely to a relationship with a single other, there would be no automatic transference to a concern with multiple others or the wider world.

Charity, for Myers, is always a relation of unequal benevolence that maintains wider inequalities rather than challenging them. For her it produces a 'real gap' from a project of associative democratic practice 'in which citizens act publicly and collaboratively in order to shape the world in which they live' (Ibid: 83). While the descriptions of charitable organisations in Myers work are somewhat narrow and ignore many of the social change, campaigning efforts of some of the charity or not for profit sector, the key point here is that the idea of a gap has a double problem. First, in proposing a space between dyadic care and any automatic care for the world, there might just as easily be a similar gap the other way around. If we only focus on care for the world and turn our collaborative efforts with others towards care for global issues (climate change, legal changes, public campaigns and so forth), there is a potential gap in how people work with each other, care for their colleagues and comrades and create the caring environments for participation that enable people to be present in these democratic practices in the first place. Put simply, we know that if interpersonal caring practices are not imbricated within the democratic practices of caring for the wider world, certain people will be left looking after the children and cooking the food, when others are marching for their rights.

The second problem is that it is wrong to see a gap, some kind of societal space, between one type of relation and another. There are not dyadic relations in one part of the world, and then associations of people caring for a particular worldly concern elsewhere. There is, to paraphrase Butler, a matrix of relations which extend from dyads, to small groups, to communities of association and back. They have strong and weak, sustaining, and oppressing points of connection, rather than being sealed discretely from each other. We need to think about networks of different, but always interconnected, caring practices which form patterns of micro and macro solidarity, with nurturing, facilitating and collaborative possibilities. There can be paternalistic practices in the relationships, but we can also point to patterns of caring that are mutually supportive which permit social participation in dignified and sometimes joyful ways. Caring for a severely disabled elder, including intimate care for bodily functions, can be done with a sense of warmth and affection, and work towards a purposeful, well lived life. It is not automatically separate from, for example, the carer's work to unionise elder care workers and her efforts to improve the conditions in privatised care homes. Touching literally and being touched affectively by a person, a situation, or an issue, traverse relations in all directions and in unpredictable patterns. There is no gap, but different strengths of caring practices and felt responses. A bond with your life partner might form the core strength sustaining your joint political work for refugees, which might be enabled because another family member cares for your parent. Being aware of the complexity of these care networks and attending to the inequalities of participation they either allow or counter, means dyadic, networked, and world-focused care cannot be packaged separately or placed into neat hierarchies of importance. Caring for an oil spill might be valid and worthy, but if action against it fails to note that it takes global majority women caring for the children of protestors to allow them to attend their rallies, then the ethical failure is obvious.

The type of networks of care suggested here correspond to Sevenhuijsen's notion of 'caring solidarity' (148) where the matrix of interconnections cannot be reduced to its component parts. In her words, this is needed not 'because the "needy" are dependent on the solidarity of the "strong", or because the "strong" need to defend themselves against the looming threat of society's corruption by the "needy" [...] but because everyone in different ways and to different degrees needs care at some point in their lives' (2003: 147). Here we have a vision of care that is facilitative in that it seeks in different ways to make lives and different forms of participation within and between communities possible. It is a restatement of Paul Gilroy's search for a 'cosmopolitan solidarity from below' (2004: 89) that for him is a more 'intimate conception of solidarity' (Ibid: 86), as opposed to one defined only as a form of public action between groups, organisations, or even nations. While solidarity is a positive ambition for these relations of care, and in terms of care aesthetics, it is the affective nature of their practice that will be the focus, for care ethics it is important to emphasise Sevenhuijsen's final line here that *everyone needs care at some point in their lives*. If relations of care are an ontological given, the extended point is that ongoing dependency is inevitable, and not something to deny or decry. Caring relations are something that all rely on, and caring solidarity is an interhuman need, even if it can be a struggle to provide or is undermined by multiple different types of inequality.

Interdependence

Even where caring solidarity does not thrive, the interdependent nature of human life is still apparent. Care ethics, therefore, insists on recognising networks of care which place people as 'inextricably interdependent' (Kittay, 2015: 57) rather than starting from individual autonomy as a social good, or aspiration for human flourishing. This approach echoes the previous chapter where the ambition for an autonomous artist or aesthetic realm was similarly questioned. It is not that individual freedom or the demand for human autonomy is framed as a negative ambition, it is that claims for autonomy or descriptions of freely chosen human behaviour, conceal the caring relations that make them possible. Independence is, therefore, largely a fiction. In Virginia Held's words, 'moralities built on the image of the independent, autonomous, rational individual largely overlook the reality of human dependence and the morality for which it calls' (2006: 10). Demanding free action in the public sphere or validating it as the high point of human achievement, is frequently based on a failure to recognise the caring infrastructures that make that presence possible in the first place. Care ethics points out that these denials are often claims of an assumed-to-be rational 'man' who refuses to recognise the multiple dependencies that enable his freedom of passage into public life. Joan Tronto argues that the capacity of individuals to 'ignore certain forms of hardships that they do not face' (1993: 121) is a form of 'privileged irresponsibility' (2013: 64). This position is not one of gender essentialism but one that is asking 'how and why hegemonic forms of masculinity licence men's neglect of caring responsibilities' (Robinson, 2011: 79). In pointing out the reality of interdependence, noting for example that attending a theatre workshop demands someone provides safe transport, is not the same as saying interdependency itself is inevitably a network of equality. While we criticise the fact that, in Judith Butler's words, 'neoliberal rationality demands self-sufficiency as a moral ideal' (2015: 12) describing the inevitable dependency of social life where all depend on relations of care for survival, also accepts that 'dependency, though not the same as a condition of subjugation, can easily become one' (Ibid: 21). The ambition of a care ethical standpoint must be to struggle for a version of interdependency where the webs of support are diverse, dynamically responsive and organised to overcome inequalities between groups and communities. While Catriona MacKenzie and colleagues argue that this should be reframed as a form of 'relational autonomy' that accepts dependency as a given but still values personal autonomy as a vital aspect of human fulfilment (2013: 22), the perspective here is that we need to 'unlearn (the) denial of dependency' (Sevenhuijsen, 2003: 19) and see instead that a desire for control or agency in one's life is nourished by and embedded within a matrix of facilitative care. This type of care might be hardly noticeable, and perhaps should be somewhat quiet or unobtrusive, but it should not be denied nor should those people, systems, or structures that provide it, be devalued. So, while facilitative care might be found in the appropriate wheelchair enabling travel, the home care that makes a working life possible, or the signer who ensures a hearing-impaired student is able to participate fully in a class, each have a sensory shape and feel. Following the approach to aesthetics outlined in the previous chapter, *Care Aesthetics* argues that these practices should be seen as part of the core, aesthetic work of any project. The traveller, worker and student might be freer to participate in areas of their lives but fixing this as the achievement of autonomy creates a false dichotomy of dependent on one side and independent on the other. The approach here is to challenge a scale that moves humans from dependent to autonomous, with the unacknowledged implication that the more autonomous one is, the more fully human. This needs to be replaced with a recognition of varying care needs of all, which change over time and according to different circumstances, and which permit different forms of participation in varying aspects of people's lives. A collaborative or solidarity ethos to care, demands that we appreciate, enhance, and improve the multiple and situation responsive types of care that enable individuals and communities to thrive – and in terms of the socially engaged arts these should be embedded in a project and not simply the support structure to it. Acknowledging interdependency can be intertwined with a demand that we have the facilitating mechanisms – people, systems, and structures – that permit us both to thrive with a more equal capacity to participate fully in our communities.

Embodied care

The approach so far has been to outline a networked approach to care ethics than contains dyadic relations, relations within groups and between people and their communities. Simultaneously it can include relations between people and objects, ideas and wider social concerns, and these are connected in an interdependent web that can provide opportunities for some to thrive, but also leaves many unsupported, cut off and denied adequate care for a 'livable life' (Butler, 2015: 21). It has a descriptive intent in presenting a mesh of care that might be equitable and life enhancing but also discriminatory or life threatening. However, it is also normative in seeking to offer an ethics of redress. This evaluative aspect is in an aspiration for a *care solidarity* where the diverse networks of facilitative and supportive care ensure more just social relations. As discussed above, care ethics does not formulate this as a list of rules for behaviour, but as a context-driven account of in situ practice. The metaphors of meshes, networks, and matrices only work to an extent in this analysis, and vitally for an argument for care aesthetics, they need to be understood as embodied, affective interrelations. Care aesthetics emphasises that this is an account of bodies acting and responding to each other, in particular cultural, social, economic, and political contexts. Twigg's use of the term 'bodywork' cannot be forgotten when the focus shifts to larger networks of practice, as it also describes multiple bodies responding to each other. She demonstrates the diversity of these activities in the following, where *bodywork* includes:

> [the] medical, therapeutic, pleasurable, aesthetic, erotic, hygienic, symbolic. It encompasses a range of practitioners: doctors, nurses, careworkers, alternative practitioners, hairdressers, beauticians, masseurs, sex workers, undertakers
>
> *(2000: 389).*

While the differences and similarities between these roles are discussed in Chapter 4, the point to emphasise here is that there is an embodied aspect of care whether it happens across large scale communities, in places such as hospitals or schools, or in micro, more intimate one-to-one practices. While Bowden in her work on parenting (2008: 29 onwards) and Sevenhuijsen in her account of 'social practices of moral deliberation' consider care as a form of 'storytelling', the argument for care aesthetics will be that this is too narrow a formulation and we need to consider the affective, physical, hands-on practices of care, as well as the narrative, perhaps more verbal, aspects. The importance of the body for care ethics, to be discussed below, has been most fully developed in the work of philosopher Maurice Hamington, particularly in his book *Embodied Care* (2004).

While Noddings early work clearly had an affective or sensory register for the experience of caring relations, where it was the 'sense of connectedness' or 'combination of excitement and serenity' that sustained them, (2013: 144),

Hamington has more firmly outlined a case that care ethics offers a 'foundation of morality rooted in our body and our bodily practices' (2004: 5). This is, of course, crucial for the case here for an aesthetics of care, as the co-created experience of a caring relationship relies on embodied skills, the sensations of the moment as it is realised between people and the shape the experience takes across time. It is worth quoting Hamington at length here as his account of the *habits of the body* leans heavily towards the concept of care aesthetics being developed here. For him, care is 'a complex intertwining of caring habits (embodied practices of interaction), caring knowledge (the embodied understandings instantiated through habits), and caring imagination (extrapolations from embodied knowledge to understand situations beyond our immediate experience and to imagine caring courses of action)' (2004: 12). There is a clear sense of a creative capacity of an individual here, as they draw on skills, imaginative resources, and embodied awareness of the needs of a situation. This, I would argue, is an aesthetic or craft repertoire drawn on to enhance the care enacted. The extension to be made from this is twofold. First, as the definitions of aesthetics in the previous chapter suggested, there is an in between quality of an aesthetic experience that materialises between object and person, or participant and other, that means we cannot only see aesthetic competence lying within one person and being realised through his or her capacity alone. This was also the point made about the intersubjective nature of touch above. It is the combination of a person with the capacities of another or the way the situation responds or feeds back into the moment, which determines the aesthetic contours of the event. The embodiment here is well described, but we must also offer an account of the other bodies, so embodiment is not only located in the sensory, body capacities of the one doing the caring. Hamington, of course, recognises this as he draws on the work of Merleau-Ponty to describe a 'synchronicity of habitual caring' that 'develops between bodies' (Ibid: 51) in a pattern that is as much 'intercorporeal' (Ibid: 55) as singularly corporal. The second extension is to pluralise this account of embodiment, so that the *intercorporeal* is not only dyadic, but realised between complex communities of care, or networks of care practices. *Bodywork* is undertaken in the multiple caring interactions drawn from habits of numerous bodies and is exhibited between many people across the dynamic social contexts of life. It is therefore as possible to speak of the bodywork at play within an institution at moment in time, as it is to focus on the bodywork between an individual meeting the needs of her or his intimate other.

From embodied care to care aesthetics

The step from an account of care ethics that notes its embodied character to one that makes the case for care having an important aesthetic element, is somewhat straightforward. Certainly, in Hamington's work this is a clear implication in that he notes 'there is very little in contemporary care ethics literature that addresses the role of aesthetics and imagination' (2011: 125) but equally he is convinced that 'care is an aesthetic activity' (2015: 278). My account here is indebted to Hamington's extended analysis of both care as an aesthetic or artful activity and then the role of the arts in educating for 'caring performances' (2010: 689). Before confirming the connection, however, it is important to mention that as a field care ethics has more traditionally been cautious about aesthetics, and at times it has exhibited strong suspicion of any claim for its relevance. These doubts will be outlined here, alongside a discussion of how bodywork has been presented as *aesthetic* in a way that suggests it is a potentially problematic aspect of caring behaviour. These comments will then lead onto a discussion of the idea of the performance of care below.

Noddings' ground-breaking early work on care ethics was hostile to aesthetics as she separated it from the care of people and understood it only as the realm of care for 'things and ideas' (2013: 21). For her it was potentially a dangerous distraction from proper attention to the needs of others, as carers were absorbed in objects or ideas to an extent that they forgot the suffering of actual people. Her analysis of what she labels 'aesthetic caring' was a 'special problem' due to how care ethics could be 'enhanced, distorted, or even diminished' by it (Ibid). I will deal below with the difference in care for people and care for objects, but the point here is that for Noddings care for objects (and ideas) was understood as aesthetic in orientation and as such a diversion from an ethical consideration of the needs of people. As will be clear from Chapter 1, this is a particular understanding of aesthetics, and simultaneously a perspective that is over reliant on dyadic, inter-human care as the 'proper' relation with which care ethics is concerned. Following the previous chapter's argument, aesthetic experience does exist between people and does not only materialise in a person's appreciation of the beauty of an object. Interestingly, the attempt to create a clear distinction between ethics and aesthetics starts to break down as Noddings notes the similarities between certain features of an artist's work and the practice of care. She argues the 'receptivity characteristic of aesthetic engagement is very like the receptivity of caring' (Ibid: 22) and that the creativity of the artist 'is present to the work of art as it is forming: listening, watching, feeling, contributing' (Ibid). While she is still suggesting that turning one's capacity for receptivity towards an artistic activity might diminish one's interest in or time for the needs of others, there is a hint that there is a similarity in the type of attention demanded by art and caring. The case being made here is that while the focus for this attention might be different, there is a sensibility at play in the one caring and the one who is focused on an art practice, which can contribute to an aesthetic experience, and both can, therefore, be examples of an aesthetic practice.

It is not only Nodding's who expresses doubt about the ethics and the aesthetics of care being aligned. In the work of Joan Tronto there is also reluctance to accept the possibility that art making might constitute care. While this is not a dismissal of aesthetics per se, it is an assertion that 'the pursuit of pleasure, creative activity' cannot be care, again suggesting a limited understanding of the different contexts in which art making takes place, and a failure to recognise the potential of valuing care skills as sensory or craft practices (1993: 104). While Tronto does endorse the view that 'creative activities can be undertaken with an end towards caring', ultimately, she insists that 'the pursuit of pleasure, creative activity [...] [t]o play, to fulfil a desire, to market a new product, or to create a work of art, is not care' (Ibid). As this book hopes to demonstrate, care aesthetics can be located both in art projects and care services, and in those initiatives that blur the boundary between them. The argument here is that creative activities can be done with an ambition towards caring, and conversely care activities can be done with a creativity and aesthetic sensibility. The account of Tronto is limited because of a particular understanding of what a work of art can be, and an inability to imagine caring relations as artful. Art making is again focused on 'production' (Ibid) and is thus a distraction from care, and not potentially a component of it. Significantly, Tronto qualifies her disavowal of 'creative activity' with a footnote which suggests that dance therapy might be a place where art making itself is purposefully caring, and in doing so, she opens up the very site of community-based, relational art making that will be a focus of this edition, specifically developed in Chapter 3 (Ibid: 204n).

While Hamington has suggested there is 'very little in contemporary care ethics literature that addresses the role of aesthetics and imagination' (2011: 125), the comments above indicate that it is perhaps more appropriate to say that there is either a limited understanding of aesthetics or a suspicion of it. A more extended analysis of the aesthetic qualities of care has taken place in the social care literature, for example in the work of Christina Buse and Julia Twigg on the 'materiality of dress' in the context of dementia care (2018). While Chapter 4 deals more specifically with examples of health care practices and their aesthetics, their work is important to touch on here as it illustrates some of the limitations with how care and aesthetics has been linked to date. Their account is a sympathetic analysis of the process of dressing and the tactile relations that emerge in the activity of getting residents ready for each day. They demonstrate how at its best this can be an attentive interaction where a carer responded sensitively to a 'person's embodied biography and personal aesthetic, rather than imposing a homogeneous appearance' (Ibid: 346). The touch and intimate process of dressing became a responsive and tender process of tuning into the needs of the elderly patient. The dynamic to note here, however, is that the analysis again locates the aesthetic primarily in the visible impact of the dressing, to the extent that 'the aesthetics of care' became a 'visible indicator of care quality' (Ibid: 341). The consequence is that in being an outward sign of the quality of care that a resident was receiving, the dress was the subject of scrutiny from senior staff or family members. It became a surrogate that reflected on the work of the carers, or to put it in more theatrical language, it was an activity that was aware of its audience. If care ethicists have specified the carer-to-cared-for dyad as a vital relation in care practice, the focus here on care quality introduces the care witness, a third figure, who can be a crucial arbiter in care relations. A potential problem is that the dressing of a patient in a care home might shift from a relation of *engrossment* in her or his needs, to one that is focused on how other's will interpret the way she or he is presented. Buse and Twigg summarise this issue by valuing a close analysis of the material and embodied relations surrounding dressing, but they also note that it 'raises dilemmas and tensions regarding the visibility and aesthetics of care' (Ibid: 349). Once again aesthetics is assumed to be defined by notions of visibility so that an *aesthetics of care* is one that is *over* dependent on attention to the outward appearance of that care. The implication being that aesthetics lacks substance because it is a surface focus done to appeal to another and not necessarily the person for whom cared is being provided. Buse and Twigg's account of the aesthetic is therefore visually-centric. Paradoxically, in the concluding part of their analysis, they do seek to reimagine care in a way that focuses on those 'relational and processual elements' (349) and in doing so, they offer a vision of care that echoes the relational and experiential version of aesthetics outlined in the previous chapter. They close their article with an appreciation of how dressing can be 'an opportunity for "being with", a time for one-to-one interaction, sensory engagement, and a practice of supporting identity' (Ibid: 350) in a statement that is, in fact, far closer to the concept of care aesthetics being proposed here. So, while we may reject the suggestion of care aesthetics as solely being concerned with *mere* appearance, a sign of virtue in the terms of Saito from Chapter 1, Buse and Twigg's attention to the bodily relations of care, touches on the practice of crafted care relations central to the case for care aesthetics being developed here.

While processual, relational, and networked care are central to the proposal for care aesthetics, the tendency noted in Buse and Twigg's article for care to be enacted with attention to the demands of an institution or for the approval of familial observers is an important one. They are introducing the idea of care being observed, or care as a witnessed practice, much like the exchange of gifts discussed in Chapter 1. This, I would argue, adds a sixth phase in the definition of care to those proposed by Tronto. So, in addition to caring about, caring for, care-giving, care-receiving and caring with, witnessing care needs to be included as an important aspect of contemporary care. It might be a detached observation as a person takes note of how a parent cares for her offspring in public that includes judgement made with anything from condescension to admiration. It can also be more intimate as in the case discussed above, where the family are the witness to how their loved one is being cared for in a home. Then it can be institutional or social where witnessing takes the form of cultures of regulation and accountability. Witnessing care brings in issues of surveillance, community concern, economic relations, and the monitoring or evaluation of practice. Care witnessed is, of course, the corollary of care performed, and for a book which is concerned, particularly in the following chapter, with care and the arts, it is important to note the significance of the different uses of this term. First, 'performance' can have an implied diminutive, as is the case in the Buse and Twigg article, so it suggests care as *mere* performance, solely for the benefit of witnesses with limited depth and only surface quality. In this usage the appearance of care for its audience is more important that the impact on the person cared for, and there is an inherent criticism in that it is done *only for appearances* (and 'appearance' is taken up again in Chapter 4's discussion of emotional labour).

Performed care, however, can have a broader less diminutive sense. It draws attention to the fact that the practice of care is done within a network of expectations, institutional and personal norms, that impact on how that practice is undertaken. External surveillance can affect the style of care practice, so that it is shaped partly by the exigencies of the context. This could be a micro sensitivity to the watching eyes of a parent as a teacher works with a child, but it can also be a nurse constrained by the complex demands of accountability processes that structure her every interaction with a patient. The performance here might be embodied comfortably by the carer to the extent that it becomes effortless, or it might cause dis-ease and feel like a distortion that fails the actual needs of the cared-for. Taking account of the pressure of that external demand can warp the practice away from the needs expressed by a patient, or the desire for professionally ethical practice on the part of the carer. Discerning the boundaries of external pressure and where it meets personally embodied training and the demands from the one to be cared for is of course difficult. Performances of care are both responses and repetitions. Performance is part of the continuity of a care practice, and part of an iterative process that always is accounting for the multiple demands made upon it. Saying that care is performed suggests that it is a constructed practice, and one made within the demands of the present in which it occurs. In the words of Hamington, 'the performance of care does not begin and end with a particular act of kindness' but designates a process that includes 'dramatic rehearsal, a habituation of going out and learning about others' (2015: 288). It is a performance caught within the habits and expectations of all people involved and the institutional or social context in which it takes place.

Hamington's view of 'care as performance' is a positive account of a *'political embodied performance, every iteration of which has the potential to contribute to our dynamic sense of moral identity'* (Ibid: 279. Italics in original). It is 'not about making art but about being artful' so that a 'performative theory of care does not suggest that caregivers are artists in the sense of having exceptional genius or in terms of end products, but it does suggest that caregivers are artists in terms of being aesthetically attuned to the bodies, actions, and relations of themselves to others' (Ibid). While this focus on the artful nature of care practice is exactly the concern of care aesthetics, I would qualify this perspective by noting that performances of care can also be situated within disciplining networks of micro witnessing or more macro surveillance. This is a parallel argument to that developed by Arlie Hochschild in her work on emotional labour, and how staff manage the appearance of the emotional practices demanded by their work (2003, 2012). The overlap between care aesthetics and emotional labour is taken up more directly in Chapter 4, where using emotional labour to frame the practice of care workers is compared to the emphasis provided by care aesthetics. The idea of performances of care, as understood here, may have a strong normative intent that is documenting the positive care-filled performances that develop through rehearsal and embodied habit, where a dynamic sense of moral identity can be developed in the words of Hamington. However, the institutional and cultural contexts of care can restrict the capacities of care workers and constrain their performances, so that they become perfunctory or attuned to demands that singularly fail the needs of the people who should be the focus of their practice. Rehearsing for caring behaviours may contribute to a positive ethical practice, but the iterative, responsive nature of a performance means that there are also likely to be competing, situation responsive constraints. This includes opportunities for astounding or unpredictable care done *in spite of* circumstance, in a way that demonstrates some carers' ability to perform against the grain of expectation. However, at times circumstances constrain so acutely that the performance response seems closer to neglect. If one context permits and enables a life changing care practice, including endorsement through the affirmative witnessing of it, another might demand technically competent but utterly cursory practice that *performs* but only by meeting the most basic of needs. Care aesthetics aims to account for the experience of care at an embodied level, focused upon how individuals and groups within certain contexts might create caring practices that develop more just social relations. However, it also suggests care is an iterative process that may be offered in ways that constrain or even reduce people's capacity to live well.

The politics of care aesthetics

While I suggest above that witnessed care might be conducive to encouraging dignified caring behaviours, there are multiple contemporary contexts which mitigate against this. An institutional culture might invite attention to anything but the forms of care needed for people to lead 'livable lives'. Twigg notes, for example, how 'managerial accounts' disembody care (2000: 392), Philips argues that certain types of setting ensure that care becomes 'regulated and formalized rather than spontaneous' (2007: 2), and Sevenhuijsen dismisses bureaucratic structures that impact negatively on care practices (2003: 19). These are constraints that shape the performances of care, at times ensuring carers practice more for a managerial expectation than what the cared-for or carer believe to be important. Care can be prescribed in procedures valued for their technical correctness or speed of delivery, rather than the intimacies of embodied connection they create. Care performances in these contexts are a vital location for any analysis of the ethics of care practice, but also politically significant as they can be supportive of or resistant to inequalities associated with experiences of care. An over managerial environment that results in limited or barely adequate care, can also be one that elicits surprisingly dynamic caring responses. Even at a micro level, acts of caring solidarity can find space in these seemingly restrictive environments and can be steps taken against the inequities that are prevalent in them. Sevenhuijsen argues that countering managerialism, or care bureaucracies, is a narrow form of the politics of care set against a broader mission to challenge the inequalities of power in caring. Here, however, I understand the factors constraining care's performance as being integrated into the complex matrices of care practices that repeat and develop across any given social context. There is not a broad or narrow disconnect. Managerialism creates the target-driven regimes that might determine the limited amount of time a homecare worker spends with an elderly person. This in turn ensures that her or his capacity to tend to them with the attention she or he aspires to, and the elder demands, is thwarted. Rather than a micro politics inferior to ones of greater concern, this is an important, and politically significant, interhuman dynamic that makes up the networks of care that structure what Virginia Held has labelled our contemporary 'Careless society' (128). The politics of care needs to be viewed as a continuity of practices, made up of multiple performances of care, that involve embodied practices in diverse interconnected settings. The action of a homecare worker maintaining attentive care *despite* the limits she works under is part of multiply interconnected political actions and not separate from political action done as part of a broader mission.

The final section of this chapter will outline a version of the politics of care that does not designate levels of importance of different types of care practice, or distinctions between caring for worldly issues against caring for another person. The argument for interdependence includes the claim that we are all constrained or enabled to different degrees by the care networks that shape our lives, and that we in turn shape. Demanding that these are facilitative, life sustaining, equitable and just can be done at the level of our intimate care of a close friend, the caring support networks in a workplace, or the care we demonstrate for the planet. And crucially one type of care is not possible without the other. Myers' writing is in danger of setting care for the world against or prior to care for each other, so that we should not focus 'on an individual's practice of care for the self or the Other' but instead on 'contentious and collaborative care for the world' (2013: 2). While care 'tethered to the practice of citizenship' (Ibid: 88) is a perfectly legitimate register for our caring practices, there is a problem here that we recreate another public-private sphere division where issues of 'proper' concern are larger scale, and we dismiss the importance of attention to the inequities of intimate relations. Care ethics and aesthetics claim that one cannot be untangled from the other. We need to be attuned to the fact that appearing in public requires a particular distribution of care to make it possible. A facilitating care is needed to open the public activity to all actors, not just the ones who have childcare needs met through personal financial security, or mobility needs met because of their health insurance and so forth. Without talking about the care inequalities that structure our lives and making this part of the politics of caring for our world, those absent will once again be those excluded through histories of class, racial and gender inequality.

Myers rightly mentions the political environment in the US as 'marked by ongoing struggles over energy policy, health care, immigration, the war in Afghanistan, and financial regulation, among many other issues' (Ibid: 93).

While these are important issues, they exclude campaigns of a different order such as violence against the LGBTQ+ community, the treatment of elderly people in care homes, or the emotional neglect of children. All these issues – and action taken by communities to challenge them – are distributed through networks of care that facilitate or prevent that action. Similarly, they are made worse through inequalities of care and the lack of attention to its aesthetic qualities when it is practiced. Attention to the quality of caring relations can be an act of care redistribution in itself, so focusing on these relations is a form of political action and not to be dismissed as less significant because it not of sufficient public scale. We need, in Bellacasa's words, not to be afraid to focus on 'on the uneventful [...] care's ordinary doings, the domestic unimpressive ways in which we get through the day, without which no event would be possible' (2017: 2053). Avoiding the hierarchy of importance, allows participation in different registers and at different sites of action. *Domestic ways* might seem unimpressive, but in fact they are the sight of immense skill, capacities and ingenuities that should not be belittled. This is exactly a register that the aesthetics of care is seeking to capture. Ensuring an elder is content and safe in their care home is often done with a sensitive attention rarely noted and created despite the economic restrictions in place. It might mean they are more able to contribute to decision-making in that context. It might mean that they are now in a better place to care for a grandchild, that in turn supports their daughter or son. Care for a child that has suffered neglect might mean they grow in their confidence to participate in their school, now more secure in the networks that support them. They might establish a peer support group in that school, that in turn ensures care solidarity for students in that context. Working with friends to ensure mobility needs are met, might ensure that all can attend the rally against a war or for the rights of a particular community. The politics of care ethics, or what Hamington broadens to call 'care theory' (212: 32), is shaped by attention to the horizontal and vertical matrices of interdependence and is attentive to the caring solidarity that both transforms lives and provides the means for further challenge to the inequalities and injustices that structure many contemporary societies.

One aspect of these interdependent relations that has been alluded to in this chapter, but not fully elaborated, is the connection between human-to-human care, and the care of non-human animals and objects. This is important because it is central to the post-humanist care ethics of writers such as Myers and Bellacasa but also because it links back to the previous chapter. The ambition of the case for an aesthetics of care in Chapter 1 sort to move aesthetic theory away from the priority given to people and object relations, specifically in relation to the dominance of the visual. It therefore proposed an aesthetics of experience that could be found in processual, human-to-human activity, and ultimately one that included aesthetics in object care without assuming that it was primary. While care in care ethics has more often been about asserting the importance of our relations with human others, relations with animals and objects, in the broadest possible sense, need to be considered as well. While a focus on the object of care was understood as a distraction by Noddings, and part of her suspicion of aesthetics, the case here is that the history of object care in the arts, and in museums in particular, is a significant part of an inclusive form of care theory. It is not the case that highly attuned capacity to care for objects, such as might be seen in the intricacies of object handling (for example Chatterjee, 2008), is immediately transferable into care for animals or humans, but the willingness to respond to the demands of the objects in our environment, or the willingness for them to be ignored or even destroyed, must be part of an understanding of a complex interdependent world. This is not a return to the dominance of care for what can be seen, but an embodied sense of being in the material world, responding to its demands on us, and being responsive to the shape and feel of the environment in which we are located and on which we are dependent. Objects that extend from our limbs, such as scalpels, brushes, or pens, are an intimate means of engaging with different worlds (see Chapter 4), where boundaries between human and non-human are blurred, and agency is distributed through interconnections between bodies and environments. This, of course, can be extended to a larger scale to include vehicles, computers, and weapons (whether swords or drones). Often these objects have been crafted by us or our predecessors but then in turn act upon the affective relations we experience within the material world. A more dynamic version of interdependency here ensures that we do not simply impress our will on the world, whether to care and repair, or neglect and damage. In the words of Bellacasa, we need to reframe Tronto's definition of care ethics from everything *we* do repair the world, to 'everything that is done [...] to maintain, continue, and repair "the world" so that all (rather than "we") can live in it as well as possible' (2017: 2800). Interactions between all elements of the material world are an ongoing process of which human agency is only one part, and the collective activity produces a 'thick mesh of relational obligation' (Ibid: 402). While there is an important lesson in humility here, so that humans are decentred from a seemingly inevitable role as world makers, the mesh metaphor should not be taken to imply that ethical responsibility for injustices or abuses is distributed equally across it. *Care's ordinary doings* must allow for particular human doings to be subject to critique. The oil spill acts on the world, and therefore is included in the mesh of interdependencies of a care-constrained society, but 'collaborative caretaking' (Myers, 2013: 87) should make demands on a human responsibility for ensuring mechanisms for adequate repair are in place.

The 'thick mesh' is human bodies, animals, objects, environments, and ideas or concepts, brought together in what geographers of care call carescapes (Bowlby et al, 2010: 247). People care about abstract ideas, peace, the nation and so forth, and these loop into how care is enacted between individuals, groups, and the contexts in which we operate. There is a politics of the distribution of care, of the economies, the inequalities of access and quality of experiences. Care ethics points to the situatedness of this politics, its particular responsiveness to moments, and rather than designating rules of behaviour, it pushes for attention to all those aspects that make life more liveable, equitable and just. This connects the micro sustenance of early life to sustaining the ecology of a planet on which we all rely. Care as practiced and embodied, as skilled capacity and a structure of relations, as a sensation of connection and a distribution of affective solidarities, needs to acknowledge that it has an aesthetic dimension. We touch and are touched by care and respond to the beauty of relationships and the joyous interactions between communities. We also know that care can be ugly or neglected, and these inadequacies of care also have an aesthetic. They are the sensory experience of living in a careless society, in a care-starved institution or a care-worn relationship. The shape, practice, and possibilities for both the positive and negative versions of care aesthetics – from its limitations to its sensuous reach – become the subject of the next chapters, as they explore care aesthetics in practice: in the world of the arts, health, and social care, and in everyday life.

Part II

Care Aesthetics in Practice

3

Careful art

Part 1 explained the concept of care aesthetics and how its constituent parts are to be defined. Part 2 will apply the concept across three chapters, dealing in turn with care aesthetics and the arts, care aesthetics and health and social care, and then finally, care aesthetics in everyday life. Each one is not simply an attempt to show how the concept works in these interconnected realms but also an exploration of how practices within these areas of social life speak back and challenge the idea. Each asks how a focus on care aesthetics develops new perspectives and new orientations for practice, and how the debates already at play in these different contexts provide new understandings for the scope of the proposal laid out in Part 1.

Introducing careful art

The title of this chapter is deliberately provocative in two senses. First using the word careful as a descriptor of art immediately draws the criticism that it must be talking about a practice that is peculiarly safe, un-risky, and maybe even dull. Careful, after all, cannot be interesting: to put careful *before* art must be condemning it to avoid all the challenge, disruption and excitement that is its hallmark. Imagine responding to a student's work with the feedback that *it was a bit careful*. So, my first provocation is that the chapter will be justifying the appropriateness of this adjective and asserting the importance of accepting carefulness as a perfectly reasonable guiding word for art making. The second provocation is the use of the generic word *art* – a sweeping term for such a broad range of practices that, it could be argued, it cannot possibly be covered within one chapter. Are we really talking about careful art that includes theatre, dance, visual art, music, film, and so on? The opening disclaimer is that, of course, the chapter will be more specific about exactly what is meant by *careful* in terms of arts practices,

DOI: 10.4324/9781003260066-6

and then which arts, at which point in the history of contemporary art, are being discussed. That said, even with greater precision in mind, I do want to challenge the perspective that sees *taking care* in art practice as something immediately constraining, and necessarily a taming influence on the power of art. Similarly, I want to ask how a dedication to carefulness might in fact speak to arts practices in the widest range of traditions and contexts. As my own background is in socially engaged performance and applied theatre, these will inevitably get particular attention, but the immediate signal here is that careful art might be a framework for understanding multiple arts practices, perhaps applicable to a knitting circle, a pottery studio, and a youth theatre workshop. Of course, there are radical differences and implications for bringing care to art making in these varied contexts, but the aim is to explore the connections that carefulness, and ultimately the idea of care aesthetics, permits between them.

One reason the chapter refers to 'arts' and is not called Applied Theatre and Care Aesthetics is that arguably the boundaries of applied theatre itself have shifted in the last few years and there has been a considerable interaction with other contemporary arts practices. Andy Lavender refers to an 'age of engagement' (2016: 21) and if we take this together with art curator Nicolas Bourriaud's argument for a *relational aesthetics* through which many artists now take 'being-together as a central theme' (2002: 15), we notice overlapping fields concerned with forms of experience and participation operating across boundaries of fine art, applied theatre, socially engaged arts, and everyday culture. Lavender notes 'works that might previously have been encountered only in applied theatre contexts have appeared on different stages' (2016: 27) and I would argue while motivations might differ, there are now points of comparison to be made across different practices of contemporary performance and related arts. Jen Harvie makes the same point when she notes that the 'boundaries between contemporary "applied" and "fine" art practices, and between art and activism, are very porous' (2013: 1), suggesting that terms such as care, which might be more familiar in applied theatre, now by necessity become important considerations in other areas of art practice.

Nicola Shaughnessy helpfully points to the etymology of 'applying' by noting that 'implicit in this terminology is the concept of "care"' (2012: xiv), and the argument here extends this to insist that caring and carefulness now become concepts that need to be drawn more systematically across a range of arts practices in our *age of engagement* to question the substance – the material, embodied acts of interaction – of which it is comprised. Grant Kester has explained a shift in aesthetic concern from the visual to 'one concerned with the generative experience of collective interaction' (2011: 24) and while I cannot claim that this is *all arts*, it is a shift that, this chapter will argue, leads to a demand for greater attention to the care ethics and aesthetics of different arts-based, interactive, and collective practices.

The performance artist Adrian Howells, who will be discussed more below, argued that 'we're living in very brutalized and unloving times' (in Machon,

2017: 19) and, therefore, these demands for new forms of engagement are not simply artistic conceits but are necessary in a society that works against interhuman intimacy. This perspective is echoed by theatre academic Alice O'Grady in her work on risk and performance, where she sees the interest in participation, commenting particularly on the work of performance artist Marina Abramović, as a product of 'a thirst for intimacy and presence that is perhaps missing from other aspects of our daily life' (2017: 33). It could be argued, therefore, that our *age of engagement*, one responding to a need for new forms of collective interaction is a product of a social life where these forms of close and meaningful experiences are diminished. Whether the blurring of boundaries between applied theatre and other areas of artistic practice, across the broader fields of 'social practice' or 'socially engaged art', is a result of new dynamics in an over-individualised social world, would however be difficult to prove. The point to emphasise is that the age of engagement does not only mean that certain boundaries between the visual, performance, and other art forms are porous but also the division between the affective experience of social life and artistic practice is less clearly differentiated. Shannon Jackson has explained in her seminal book *Social Works* how we need to explore the 'artistic skills required to sustain the Life side of the supposed Art/Life binary' (2011: 29) and for this chapter the crucial word here is *supposed*. By announcing the importance of the dynamics of caring for artistic practice, the argument is that the desire to police the boundary between art making as a realm of aesthetic practice and an alternative world of the ethical and social, is unsustainable in much contemporary art practice, and is one that *care aesthetics* seeks to challenge specifically. Jackson's work brings the social support for art practice, the social systems that make it possible, to the fore to reveal infrastructures that might enable what she labels 'aesthetic conviviality' (2011: 6). While this chapter will draw on her analysis, one where 'the aesthetic infrastructure that supports the aesthetic object coincides with the exposure of the social infrastructure that supports human societies' (Ibid: 39), here there is a slightly different emphasis. It is one where the notion of the aesthetic and the social coinciding is somewhat stronger, and what differentiates infrastructure from that which it supports is less clear. The argument proposes a notion of the aesthetic integrated with the social, explained as a form of *simultaneity* in the last section of the chapter. It seeks a less distinct demarcation of that which is designated support and that which is the thing supported. Within an argument for an aesthetics located in the experience across the full duration of an art making process rather than a singular object or event, those supportive or caring systems enabling practice, are less background and more often embedded within the art project itself. Care does not enable art making here: care is part and parcel of the experience of the art itself.

Chapter 3 will outline this integrative approach to *careful art* by locating it in what has been called the *social turn* in visual and performance arts, but, in anticipation of Chapter 4, also noting that this has missed a complementary cultural turn in aspects of the social. In many ways this is a conversation with the established arts and health movement, linked also to Phil Hanlon and Sandra Carlisle's notion of the 'fifth wave in public health' (2016: 20), which will be touched on briefly below. The chapter includes accounts of practice, some encountered personally and some drawn from descriptions of others, that allow us to catch glimpses of care aesthetics in different art making contexts. The final sections of the chapter will place the case for careful art into contemporary debates about the relations between art making and society, arguing for an embedded aesthetic-ethical set of practices that draw on the theories of aesthetics from Chapter 1 and care from Chapter 2. Careful art is presented as a product of human inter-dependence, relational experience and the importance of processes undertaken over time. It draws from a desire to trust rather than confront audiences, produce dramaturgies of care rather than discomfort and a simultaneity in our considerations of ethical and aesthetic matters.

Several commentators have noted how the 21st century has accelerated what is called the 'social turn' in the visual and performing arts. Jackson refers to this as a 'performative turn' which has foregrounded an interest in 'the nature of sociality' (2011: 2) and then a 'social turn' which has led to a crossing of boundaries between different art mediums, for example where theatre draws on architecture or sculpture becomes more choreographic (Ibid: 28). Lavender notes a shift that is particular to theatre and performance as practitioners 'connect more overtly with social processes' (2016: 3) and Harvie sees the turn as evidenced by an engagement with 'other delegated workers' rather than solely with audiences (2013: 5). Importantly, these authors are offering descriptions rather than critiques of this development, which for them is not necessarily seen as a threat to the integrity of the artistry of these practices. Others are noticeably less sanguine presenting the movement which results in the 'embedding of the artists in the social field' (Bishop, 2012: 205) as one that replaces our 'rightful' focus on aesthetics with 'sociological discourse' (Ibid: 17). These debates will be discussed in more detail later with the ambition to dismiss the concerns less by challenging the effect of a sociological discourse on art making processes, and more by suggesting that we are mistaken if we see this as an abandonment of aesthetics. While theatre scholars such as Rat Western might see these shifts as producing a 'stultification' (2017: 185) of both the freedom and artistry of practitioners, the argument here is that the new forms of sociality that might be the ambition of the social turn have an aesthetics as well and are therefore not only governed by discourses of a sociological nature. Far from being a retreat from 'properly' aesthetic concerns as artists are 'obliged to step in' where 'social agencies have failed' (Bishop, 2012: 38), the argument for careful art, and care aesthetics more broadly is that we need to challenge the distinction made between 'Art/Life' and make the case that Jackson's 'aesthetic conviviality' might be a descriptor for activities across different realms of human experience. It, therefore, troubles what might be straightforwardly referred to as artistic and social realms, and the 'turn' might in fact be a shift to new contexts which are themselves rich with aesthetic practices rather than the aesthetic-less wastelands that some might assume.

While this perspective is sympathetic to Grant Kester's account of the 'postindustrial' artist who 'must now create alternative models of sociality to challenge the instrumentalizing of human social interactions characteristic of a postindustrial economic system' (2011: 30), its emphasis is different. Here the argument is that these models of sociality have an aesthetic sensibility already, and artists may contribute, magnify, or expand the felt experience of that sociality, but it is not a burden that only they are able or assumed to carry. Where this chapter does focus on the work of artists and arts projects, the orientation of the book as a whole is to challenge the narrowness of Kester's category of the postindustrial artist. Here the suggestion is that we need to expand our vision of who may be included and reimagine a broader category of postindustrial worker who has a role in augmenting the aesthetic richness of our communal sociality. The argument of care aesthetics is that carers (in formal, informal, and everyday settings) when given proper support and acknowledgement can and do *create alternative models of sociality*. They are often highly skilled aestheticians and therefore play a vital role in making life more convivial. Jackson explains that her work focuses on 'trained visual artists as they turn to performance to expand their practice and engage wider systems of social and aesthetic support' (2011: 41) and while there may be a similar focus on trained artists and their projects in this chapter, it is important to emphasise that this is only part of a wider argument that suggests we should also draw attention to, and more consistently learn from, those other workers who are also involved in maintaining social and aesthetic support in diverse, widely distributed social-aesthetic settings. For *Care Aesthetics*, these are the health professionals, home care workers, teachers, and everyday carers who will be the focus of Chapters 4 and 5. The book is arguing that artists have a role in developing aesthetically rich and life sustaining caring communities, but they need to budge over a bit, and share the limelight with a whole host of others. This point is further touched on in the work of Adrian Howells, particularly at the end of the chapter.

Before starting to look at practices in detail, it is important to note how much the approach in *Care Aesthetics* is in debt to the history, scholarship, and practice in the field of arts in health. This area has developed a strong degree of support in policy circles, particularly in the UK after the publication of the All Party Parliamentary Group report in 2017 called '*Creative Health: The Arts for Health and Wellbeing*' (APPG, 2017). It is impossible to characterise the diversity of practices documented in that publication here, but important to note that many of the examples below could be included in this or similar reports. An example of the breadth of contexts and approaches can also be glimpsed in the book edited by Stephen Clift and Paul Camic, called '*Creative Arts, Health and Wellbeing*' (2016). One key difference here, however, is the desire to trouble the distinction between the two contexts that surround the simple word 'in', and this is by no means an approach alien to many arts *in* health practitioners themselves. Here rather than a straightforward focus on artists working in health contexts, the approach is that health contexts already develop aesthetic experiences across multiple practices (some developed by those designated health professionals and some by those designated artists). Similarly, many cultural contexts, and the practices developed within them, could be understood for their contribution to health care broadly conceived. When the theatre scholar Emma Brodinski, in her account of theatre in health and care settings, argues that 'interaction rather than co-existence is necessary if arts and health practitioners hope to explore the connections between disciplines and develop new pathways', the emphasis here is to take this one step further (2010: 11). Rather than an interaction between parties that seeks proper language to describe the health care outcomes of an artistic practice, care aesthetics proposes a practical-theoretical account from which diverse practitioner groups might draw or to which they might contribute. Brodinski rightly argues for a 'common language' (Ibid: 12) but here the aim is to animate, and draw attention to, the aesthetics of the different care relations within health (and many other) settings at the same time as highlighting the caring aspects of arts practices. At best, we might find new approaches to healthy, sensorially rewarding and engaging ways of living which operate as both. This is anticipated in what Hanlon and Carlisle's 'Fifth wave of public health' where they seek 'integrative' practices that combine science, ethics, and aesthetics (2016: 23). If from their perspective, late modernity is faced more by dis-ease than what historically has been the challenge of disease, we should avoid 'reductionist studies that seek to show biomedical benefits from interventions that involve art or music' (Ibid). An alternative, for these writers, is a broader model that does nothing less than reimagine 'what it is to be fully human and live together in a healthy, sustainable, just, but also beautiful world' (Ibid). When giving examples of practices that fit this ambitious demand for a new integrated approach to public health, these writers avoid grandiose projects and chose instead for their archetypal example the simple preparation of food (a topic that is returned to in Chapter 5). It is worth quoting them in full as a prelude to the discussion that follows, as this introduces care aesthetics in practice, and shows it traversing the neat lines, between art, health, and everyday life.

> We do not eat with either science or ethics as our most prominent motivations. We eat because we get hungry – but eating is not empty of social meaning. We eat to share fellowship with friends and family. We prepare food to show love and care for others. We express our creativity when we prepare food and our appreciation when we receive food [...] we eat out of an integrated mixture of all these factors
>
> *(Ibid).*

Rather than a model that seeks to warn about the diminishing of art as it meets the social, or even a model that foregrounds support structures that might be hidden in many art practices, this integrated or simultaneous approach hopes to reveal caring possibilities in art making, and artful possibilities in caring. With this in mind, we now turn to examples of art practice: examples of careful art.

Careful art in practice

The next section starts with two examples – one part of a participatory process, and one a live performance. The chapter then continues with explorations of different areas of artistic and largely performance practice, to illustrate how different contexts can be explored through a care aesthetics framework. These examples of care aesthetics in practice then lead into a discussion of the implications of this approach for contemporary debates in the socially engaged arts. The first two are drawn from my writing on care aesthetics in the edition *Performing Care* (Stuart Fisher and Thompson, 2020).

Grandchildren of Hiroshima

In April 2015 London Bubble Theatre was working on a new performance piece in Hiroshima, Japan called *Grandchildren of Hiroshima* as part of a project to commemorate the 70th anniversary of the bombing of the city in August 1945. I have written elsewhere about the broader project (Thompson, 2017) and here will only focus on one exercise from a workshop early in the process (borrowed from the account in Thompson, 2020). I want to demonstrate how the playing of games can exhibit but then importantly practice and build an experience of care aesthetics. This was particularly important in this context, as the project was intergenerational, bringing young children into contact with elders in a programme that asked questions about how younger Japanese people could connect with the experiences of the war generation. Playing with each other became an actual moment of connecting and not just a representation of that need. Similarly, through an embodied process of playing with children, elders became reconnected to memories of themselves as children at the time of the nuclear attack.

Games within community-based theatre have numerous purposes including the sensitising of participants to their own and others' bodies, the rekindling of a capacity for and comfort with play so vital for collaborative theatre making, and to enhance an embodied sense of connection and trust with one's fellow participants. Play can be joyous, disruptive, and anarchic, as well as rule-bound, disciplinary and, of course, controlling. The intention here is not to offer a detailed analysis of play within community performance, but to argue that its relational qualities can prepare groups for attentiveness to the other, enhancing their caring capacities. While I have no doubt that games can be used to exclude and divide, the account here suggests that they can also develop a practice of inter-human care, creating in Tronto's words 'the qualities of solidarity and trust' (2015: 262) that are a crucial part of care aesthetics.

Early in one of the group's first workshops the director of London Bubble, Jonathan Petherbridge, chose an exercise that required the group to work in pairs. The participants, a mix of Japanese children, young adults, and elders, were all working on a performance piece about the experience of people on the day of the atomic bombing of Hiroshima. The exercise was broken into several stages, becoming more challenging as it progressed. The first stage required one person 'A' in the pair to rest his or her hand on the 'B' partner's shoulder and then with the other hand hold the partner's left hand gently. 'A' was then asked to guide 'B' around the space with 'B' keeping her or his eyes shut. After a short period of the pairs taking tentative – careful – steps around the space, they were asked to swap over so 'B' took on the 'A' role, and the process was repeated.

At all times, Petherbridge encouraged people both to explore the space but also ensured that the person with their eyes closed was marshalled gently around without bumping into other people or objects. After this first element of the exercise, the partners briefly discussed how they felt about it – was this safe, scary, or enjoyable? The next stage increased the challenge, and the lead partner no longer held the other's hand but just placed his or her single hand on the shoulder of their collaborator. There was the same close process of directing someone around the space, but the connection was lighter. After both had done this variant, it was changed once again, so that the lead now kept her or his hand on the shoulder only to direct movement but took it off otherwise, leaving the partner to move around the space with no contact. The hand was only returned to the shoulder to redirect, slow down or stop a person: that is, to keep them safe from the other players and obstacles in the room. The final stage changed again with the instruction for the leaders to make eye contact with other leaders and when they took their hands off a partners' shoulder, they swapped partner and moved their hand to a new shoulder. Ideally the person with their eyes closed hardly noticed the switch, as they were conducted around the room with different partners just making gentle shoulder touches to stop, turn and carefully orientate them only when absolutely necessary. In the playing, this final section lasted longest with the group quietly and relatively effortlessly allowing the walkers their space with the leaders pivoting between different individuals allowing them to explore the room safely.

This final stage was balletic as a lead partner moved stealthily around the room to catch a new person and then pirouette around another. Each needed to be minutely connected with other leaders to ensure that all remained safe, at the same time as watching closely for her or his original partner, and partners they would soon be assisting. The exercise built a particular (not of course completely unproblematic) model of care. First, there was an intimate connection to the direct partner as the person quietly led him or her around the space. Second, as the touch became lighter, there was the experience of the reciprocal nature of that touch as the person being led had to respond to the feel of the fingers and had to concentrate on the quality of the connection to understand what it sought. Finally, there was an ensemble moving in a combined act of care that shared responsibility for ensuring people could move safely around the space. In this final stage, just as a person released the touch from one person, she or he moved on to support another and the exercise built to the point where relative independence was assured by the sensation that if someone shifted too close to an edge or to a table, she or he would be retrieved by someone in the group: by a sense of collective responsibility. As the exercise developed the somewhat functional, perhaps over-protective hand-on-shoulder-hand-in-hand relationship became replaced with more relaxed, gentler movements of the eye-closed partner, coupled with the dance of care around the different partners as the others moved to support each other, balancing and shifting physically through the space with a range of movements whose objective was to ensure the collective safety of all players. And this was a display, a choreography of care, as the fluid movements had a shape and pattern: it was dance-like as one person caught another, but then moved to someone else, shifting a body around the space to ensure the network of care and support was not broken. But of course, it also was not a display, in the sense of being for someone outside the group to witness. It existed in its own right as a mutual and relational experience for the group that modelled, and built that subtle trust needed for quality ensemble work.

As I note above, there is a danger in assuming that this is a fully acceptable metaphor for an aesthetic realisation of a caring relationship. Requiring one person to close their eyes, hints at the disabling metaphor at the centre of the exercise. There is, of course, the danger of paternalism in the relationship between the carer and the 'blind' cared for, where one ultimately maintains the direction and power over the other. Care ethics is concerned with the inequalities and imbalances in caring relations as much as the potential for forging more just relations based on mutual interdependency. A response to this problem did, however, emerge here. As the exercise developed, we witnessed some surprising acts of support, for example between a smaller child and an adult, or between a teenager and an elder, and between women and men. The exercise, in fact, could be viewed as one that shifted the dynamics of interpersonal care and reassembled caring relations in ways that broke some of the expected, more familiar relations between children and elders, and between the young and the old. A trust game that was part of the process of assembling a theatre-making ensemble, thus made new forms of mutual awareness and interpersonal solidarity possible. This does not overcome the problem of power differentials that are real in this type of exercise but does show how power in care adjusts in the ways it is enacted between people over time. Care aesthetics draws attention to these dynamics through particular focus on the shifting embodied quality of caring experiences.

In this example, caring expertise – that grew through the exercise – had an artistry, a physicality and sensory quality. It was not the perhaps clumsy touch of the opening stage (which was a literal aiding of a partner and, of course, a metaphor for multiple different interpersonal relationships) that was valued, but the emergent delicate touch, release and sharing of responsibility for collective care. In a way this mirrored the shift in care ethics from one-to-one caring relationships (for example, parent to child) to more social models of caring, discussed in the previous chapter. The shift was made visible through the exercise in a process of increased difficulty, and increased focus on the collective responsibility for multiple, interrelated acts of care. Significantly for *care aesthetics*, the success of this more collective stage required the interdependent care to be valued in part, of course, for its gracefulness. A child lightly touched the shoulder of an older woman to keep her safe; a teenage girl coaxed a middle-aged man to move gently across the room. The game demonstrated that the execution of care for the other required practice, rehearsal in the theatrical sense, as well as networks of connectedness and mutual support. However, it also showed that it required craft, attention to minute differences in inter-human physicality and a sense of awareness of the body in space and its rhythms of connection to others. This was an *outcome* that was realised within the process itself and was not merely a moment of preparation for a final performance. This was not, therefore, care 'like' a dance, as if the dance were a metaphor for or representation of care. Instead, high quality care was shown in and of itself to have the aesthetic dimensions of dance – and the more graceful the dance, the higher quality the care. The exercise built the group's capacity to respond and then enabled them to enjoy dancing their care for each other.

Care aesthetics highlights this simultaneity – where art making and care taking happen at one and the same time, and where the social outcome and the aesthetic experience cannot be untangled.

Ruff

Peggy Shaw is a performance artist celebrated for her work with Lois Weaver in the duo Split Britches. Pioneers of the queer and experimental performance scene in New York in the 1960s and 1970s, they have, since the 1980s, drawn on contemporary, classical, and popular forms to create performance projects dealing with a huge range of lesbian, feminist, and other themes. Peggy Shaw, in particular, is known for her one-woman shows dealing with the many characters, stories, inspirations and personal experiences that have shaped her life. In response to her stroke in 2011, she developed a new show, *Ruff*, directed by Lois Weaver, dealing with the impact of the event on her life, her body, and her memories. It explored her subsequent recovery, her ability to recall stories and her new-found capacities and struggles. *Ruff* toured the UK in 2013 and 2014, visiting Manchester's Contact Theatre where I saw it with an audience of young people, stroke survivors and medical professionals.

Shaw took her post-stroke memory challenges as inspiration to construct a show that used monitors, green screen, and other technological memory aids, including the presence of director Lois Weaver in the audience, to enable her to move her way through its multiple sections and stories. The presence of a mobile screen on stage laid bare the support structures that are often made invisible in many performance pieces – almost in homage to a Brechtian desire to make visible the mechanics that allow the theatre to take place, and certainly a connection to the supporting infrastructures discussed in Shannon Jackson's work. They were introduced, in the words of reviewer Benjamin Gillespie, 'as though they were a supporting cast there to keep her on cue' (2013: 577). The performance had an honesty about the structures of care that were needed to make it possible, that acted as a commentary on the way theatre more usually hides how performers are enabled to appear and stay safe on stage. There was no independent autobiographical performer here, but a person acutely aware of their own vulnerability and joyously presenting the tools needed to transform that vulnerability into a live presentation. The performance was not a story of an individual with extraordinary power to overcome, but a demonstration of the inevitable need for people to draw on the care and support of others, to make, in Judith Butler's terms, 'life livable' (2015: 21). Shaw told stories from her stroke, her hospital care, her recovery, and her past, including relations with friends and family. Fragmentary accounts of tea with friends, hospital stays, and her sister's wedding, interspersed with sound from 'her band' and green screened images, built up a moving and comedic account of the stroke's impact on her life. While the monitors positioned around the front of the stage were in one sense the machinery of care, they were also, by being present with the actor, given an artistic role. They were the supporting cast or co-performers giving Shaw the care that she needed to allow the show to take an onstage form. Their presence enacted a refusal to deny the performer's dependency, and in so doing made visible something of the interdependency of all performance, and of course, all performers.

This laying bare and giving form to care in performance, however, was realised most directly in a couple of moments in the performance in Manchester which placed care at the centre of this performance, in a way that further emphasised something of the vulnerability of performers. At a couple of points in the show, Shaw looked up to ask, 'Am I in the right place?' and 'where do I go now?' From the semi-obscurity of the audience a voice was heard giving reassurance: 'yes that's right', 'you're fine', and 'yes, just there'. Director Lois Weaver was close to the front of the auditorium, ready to provide orientation and gentle guidance if the screens and other technical prompts failed to provide it. She made audible the usually unheard process of directorial guidance and signalled the care that was part of the labour inherent in it. There was something profoundly moving about this voice from the darkness. It seemed to express what was acutely present, but unspoken, in the audience; that is, an overwhelming sense of willing Shaw's success as she travelled through her complex, multi-layered story telling. During the performance, there was a nervous anticipation, almost a collective holding of breath, as those watching urged Shaw to remain in control of the show.

Weaver's words of encouragement demonstrated her care as a director for her actor, a responsibility that is by no means ubiquitous. Her interjections also voiced the audience's desire to connect with and support the unfolding narrative of Shaw's performance. The ad libs both illustrated that the facilitating human technology behind this exceptional performance was a relationship of care and in being voiced from the auditorium, she gave that care audible form. The support structure, therefore, became part of the artistry of the show – something admitted and celebrated rather than denied – and a structure that drew those in the audience into a relationship of care with the performer. Care aesthetics, here, is experienced in laying bare the relationship between audience and stage to make us all aware of the sensation of mutual regard and care that make successful performances possible. We witnessed a solo performer as a dependent person, relying on visible technologies and invisible spoken assurances.

The aesthetics of the show were not located solely in what took place on the stage, but in the sensations of mutual reliance and concern between audience and performers. In performance scholar Colette Conroy's words, it had a 'quality of reciprocal engagement' which itself 'may be thought about as aesthetic' (2017: 96). In *Ruff*, the crafted care that allowed Shaw to perform successfully became visible and part of what was appreciated about the performance. Weaver's care for Shaw in that 'you're fine' became part of the moving, care-filled quality of this piece, and spoken from within the audience, it brought those of us watching into the relationship of care that she expressed. Weaver demonstrated for the audience something of our mutual dependency. While there was a singular relationship here between performer and director, her position within the audience seemed to share that responsibility with a group of spectators who were then, in turn, called upon to care. Gillespie writes that the audience were her collaborators who 'enabled her to remain vulnerable yet protected' (2013: 577) but the show also demonstrated how this was perhaps a condition of all performance. The dance of collective care from the exercise in Hiroshima, was here the collective, heightened attention of a caring audience, drawn into a relationship with a performer who allowed her dependency to be made visible and audible. Care aesthetics was realised in an interdependent performance, where support between performer, stage devices, director and audience all combined to be central to the experience of the event.

The two examples above belong firmly to the fields of theatre and performance studies and while they should be read in relation to the vignettes used at the very beginning of the book, art making that involves relations between people are particularly productive for illustrating the development of care aesthetics in practice. The contention is, however, that exploring care aesthetics in different art forms will be vital for its development. It will be productive to explore, for example, in relation to object care in museums, in design, in sculpture, or film and these analyses will then loop back into new understandings of the possibilities of care aesthetics as a concept. For now, four additional examples will be presented. First is a return to the history of contemporary fine art in the work of Mierle Laderman Ukeles and her programme of *Maintenance Art*. Second will be theatre programmes in the context of dementia care and in particular the work of applied theatre scholar Michael Balfour. Third will be examples from dance, examining the community-based dance in the work of choreographer and performer Rosemary Lee, and the work of Israeli dancer and choreographer Yasmeen Godder. Finally, I will outline the care aesthetics that is realised in the practice of one-to-one performance work, focusing specifically on the intimate performance of the artist Adrian Howells.

Maintenance art

The artist Mierle Laderman Ukeles wrote her 'Manifesto for Maintenance Art' in 1969, as an articulation of her frustration that her attempts to work as an artist had become limited by the demands of care she was required to under-take as a new mother. She proposed that all the daily activities she undertook as a woman needed to be included as part of her art making practice. As a fine artist she asserted her right to determine what in her practice was art and what was not. So, for her, the activities of cleaning, cooking, and washing should be understood as art practices, leading her to create a proposal for an exhibition entitle CARE, where daily chores – those practices that maintained lives – were given prominence. Given this brief description, the connection in Ukeles work to care aesthetics is obvious. First, there is the clarity of her claim that daily activities should be considered as art practices and how this directly echoes Tronto's definition of care ethics as everything we do '*to maintain, continue, and repair our 'world' so that we can live in it as well as possible*' (1993: 103. Italics in the original). A care ethicist's repair of the world is presented as an art practice of everyday maintenance. *Maintenance art* is, thus, another way of presenting what is here called *careful art*. This crossover can also be noted somewhat simplisti-cally by the fact that Ukeles practice features as an important case study both in a book on the performing arts (Jackson, 2011) and a book on contemporary crises in the care system (Bunting, 2020). Bunting quotes her from 2013 in a speech about 'Maintenance Art and Care' where she argued that the work of cleaners in a museum were 'as much "culture" as the artefacts and installations in the galleries' (2020: 48). This corresponds to the case made here which would similarly argue that cleaners engage in an aesthetic practice of care. Bringing cleaning, washing, or sweeping into the gallery points to the fact that these practices, too often ignored or undervalued, have a value for the craft that it takes to undertake them and an aesthetics that should not relegate them to mere support for more important 'properly' artistic activities fit for a gallery. This is a restatement of the case for everyday aesthetics from writers such as Saito (2008, 2017) which will be returned to in Chapter 5. It also links to Jackson's project because it highlights certain social infrastructures as both vital for the artwork but also that the boundaries between support and the art object are far from stable. Ukeles felt that becoming a mother who washed, cleaned and cared had 'positioned her in a new place in the art production apparatus, on the side of the supporter and maintainer rather than on the side of the genius artist' (Jackson, 2011: 87), and by bringing her 'chores' into the gallery she highlighted the significance of those maintenance tasks and the arbitrariness of the distinc-tion between artistic and care practices. In a project where Ukeles cleaned the vitrines of display cases as an artistic act of maintenance, we see a boundary between 'the intrinsic dimensions of the art object and its extraneous forms of support, with the former falling under the purview of the conservator and the latter under the purview of the janitor' being explored (Ibid: 95).

Ukeles is an important practitioner in any argument for care aesthetics because her work revealed both a connection between repair of the world and art making, and simultaneously demonstrated how contemporary art is fraught with over policed boundaries between what is permitted as art and what is mere *chore*. That said, there are two points to make where my analysis diverges from Jackson and where we need to question some of the assumptions that are contained within this practice. The first is the power by which her maintenance work is designated art. Jackson writes that 'she decided to name her daily chores [...] "maintenance art"' (Ibid: 85) suggesting that in her act of naming, by making the claim, they became considered as part of her art practice. She was already an artist, and she wanted the new routines of child and home care that were taking a huge proportion of her time included within her 'art' practice. While it is welcome for care practices to be highlighted in this way, the perspective here is that they do not become art because or when they are named as such by an artist. Care has an aesthetic already and while many of the chores listed by Ukeles might struggle to be understood as craft, her comment on the cleaners in the 2013 speech quoted by Bunting, demonstrates that she does view the work as already involving an aesthetic before it is highlighted as such. Care aesthetics would argue that we should not wait for the act of naming done by an artist before accepting the potential for multiple care and maintenance practices to be noted for their aesthetics (and whether they are or are not legitimately 'art' is, therefore, of lesser concern).

My second point, linked to this first, is about the power of the gallery in her work. We need to ask whether Ukeles figures as a type of Duchamp of care, relocating maintenance in the gallery space and making it art because the conventions of the art space overdetermine what is placed within it. It becomes art, like Duchamp's urinal, as it is placed in a context that labels that which is displayed within it as art. While this would be an over simplistic characterisation of her work, there is a slight danger in presenting her work as a 'gesture' (Jackson, 2011: 95) it becomes a commentary on the invisibility of the support structures that permit art making, rather than an argument that these acts of maintenance are actually, inside or outside the gallery, aesthetic activities themselves. Ukeles work in the early manifesto and then her later work as Artist in Residence at the New York State Sanitation Department, provides an exemplary case for bringing aesthetic attention to acts of care and repair: to maintenance. She is, therefore, a leading candidate for early pioneer status of care aesthetics. However, the takeaway from her work emphasised here is the way she as an artist revealed the aesthetics embedded in care activities, not that they were merely framed as or named as art to make a point about their invisibility. Care can be *artful*, it has an aesthetic, in or out of the gallery.

Art in dementia care

If Ukeles' work was a trailblazer for debates about the relations between art and care, the next three examples provide more contemporary accounts of care aesthetics in practice. First, there will be a brief analysis of the many different artistic projects happening with people with dementia, where the care setting creates an opportunity to examine the integration of care and art in a particularly challenging context. The second, will be projects in the field of community dance where the art of dancing together, and in particular holding or touching others, comes to the fore. The final example is the practice of one-to-one performance where the importance of intimacy both in performance and by extension in our daily lives will be discussed.

It is beyond the scope here to provide a comprehensive overview of the dynamic and changing field of arts and dementia care. There are expert books by David Amigoni and McMullan (2019), Anne Basting (2020), Janet Gibson (2020), and Sheila McCormick (2017) that provide case studies and overviews of a field that has developed hugely as the awareness of the complexity and prevalence of dementia has become more widespread. The emphasis here is how a framework of *careful art* in relation to dementia and the care homes in which many elders live, points to the way that artists have shifted from bringing their skill set into the social context, and adapting to the demands they faced, to a dynamically integrative practice where the art activity itself is part of the delivery of high-quality care. At its best, an art initiative within a care home, whether music, storytelling, movement, or visual art, is how residents with dementia have their capacities endorsed and extended, and the quality of their lives enhanced. Anne Basting's book *Creative Care* (2020) is perhaps the most telling example where an artistic intervention in a care home means being in the moment with elders, accepting them for who they are, and creating with them. It necessarily presents an account of creativity in these contexts being a caring practice, and care needing the creative impetus of artists. What the idea of care aesthetics seeks to point to in the exemplary programmes of work as described in Basting's book is that it is through the intensity of experience developed in a finely tuned creative act of care, that the profound impact on the person and the institution in which they are living, appears to be made. Basting shows how it is often, but not always, the work of artists that shape and expand that affective experience.

Michael Balfour has illustrated this focus on experience, what he calls 'pausing to be with someone in the moment' (2019: 95), as a care aesthetic practice which itself is both a challenge to certain more perfunctory forms of care and to the more usual orientation of practices of socially engaged arts. His account of a long-term initiative with participants with mid- to late-stage dementia 'challenged many of the assumptions and intentions of art with a social intent, questioning and re-phrasing these into an ethics and aesthetics of care' (Ibid: 93). What we have in his and his colleague's work, therefore, is not an account of arts in dementia care, but an account of the importance of the aesthetics of care, to which artists, and carers, contribute. Balfour's description of a key observation from his study was the importance of 'really sitting with the joy/pleasure of a moment of shared connection' (Ibid: 95) and again this is an exemplary case of the language of care aesthetics illuminating the sensations of the moment without emphasising a boundary between artistic and social context. The concept of 'the moment' will be touched on in the chapter that follows in an account from dementia-focused nursing studies, but for now the practice outlined by Balfour's case study, and other practices by artists working in dementia care settings, provide important examples of careful art. In Basting and Balfour's work, we see accounts of arts practices in demanding contexts becoming seamlessly integrated in the quality of care provided. Balfour and his colleagues saw this as 'disruptive' of 'task-orientated care' (Ibid) and he is making, therefore, a measured criticism of the limitations in many homes, constrained as they are by multiple economic, social, and political factors. Balfour's project, in a comparable way to those documented by other scholars, provided training from artists to care home workers in attempts to integrate artistry into the care setting and provide a means for sustaining the impact of their work. The questions from a care aesthetics perspective would be how 'training' might recognise the aesthetics of the care that is already provided by those workers, and second, how in the longer term we might develop a care home culture where the high-quality aesthetic experiences of care become part of a daily expectation, with or without the artists present (a perspective echoed in the work of Luke Tanner, 2017 on cultures of touch in dementia care).

Arts in dementia care settings, therefore, illustrate two significant points for a chapter on careful art. First, care aesthetics importantly interacts with institutional care cultures, and might be a powerful way of conceptualising a meeting point for the quality of care and simultaneous quality of an arts provision, so that we argue for a more seamless practice, rather than one based on the separateness of artists and carers. Second, care aesthetics becomes a critical concept when used in relation to institutions and specific care contexts. It both provides a means to point to the aesthetically rich moments of interaction between carers and, in these examples, residents, but simultaneously, it could be used as a means for pointing to the austere nature of some care home practices, referred as the 'aesthetics of deprivation' in the work of arts and health researcher Hilary Moss and O'Neil (2014: 1032) (see further discussion in Chapter 4). Care aesthetics is, thus, both a tool of analysis but also a critique of the poverty of some examples of care practice.

Community dance

If the previous section sought to illustrate that care aesthetics might operate within a particular context, here the focus is on how it might be understood in relation to form. Dance is chosen because choreographers and dance scholars note how collaborative practice in this medium, particularly in relation to community-based dance, focuses on care of dancers and participants as a necessary means to success, and as the shape of the very bodily expressions that constitute the art (Hamera, 2011). As Fiona Bannon argues in her work on ethics and dance, echoing the language of care ethics, in dance 'attention is given to the manner of dialogic relations experienced during the creation of a work' (2018: 18). Lifting a body is done carefully for the well-being and protection of the dancers, but that careful lift is also the source of the aesthetic experience for both those dancing and those witnessing the dance. Care here does not, in Western's words, 'stultify' the aesthetic, therefore, it is a constituent part of it. In an extended analysis of a performance between professional dancers and their fathers called 'Dad Dancing: Reclaiming Fatherly Grooves' in 2014, Helen Nicholson notes this exactly when she argues that 'the intimate relationships glimpsed on stage blurred distinctions between the social, the artistic and the personal' (2017: 117). It is the capacity of community dance to make this blurring possible that is the focus of this section.

Rosemary Lee is a British based dancer and choreographer, trained at the Laban Centre, who has been producing dance pieces of different scales with professional and non-professional dancers for over 30 years. Demonstrating why she is important for a discussion of care aesthetics, Bannon describes her as a 'shaper of choreographic relations' with a 'diligent ethic of care' (2018: 195). In 2009, she created a piece of work called Common Dance, with the company Dance Umbrella, for the London Borough of Greenwich's Borough Hall. It included a small group of professional dancers alongside over 40 non-professionals, aged eight to eighty-three, and is discussed by Lee in an interview by theatre scholar Martin Welton (2013) and by theatre scholar Nicola Hatton, in her analysis of *slow practice* in applied theatre (2019: 99–100). What I want to highlight here is how for Lee the production, from rehearsal to performance, was an exercise in 'negotiated togetherness', or in Welton's words 'an approach to performance that entreats audiences and dancers alike, to pay attention to one another, with care' (Ibid: 2368). In one sense, this operates much like Jackson's supporting infrastructures, so that her work, in the words of Caoimhe McAvinchey 'models a politics of collaboration' (2013: 280), providing an ethical framework that positions her process as a social practice. This then invites the viewer and the participants 'to attend to each other' in a way that is crafted 'through principles of intimacy, care, equity and justice' (Ibid: 359). Lee is important for the debate here, however, because her practice permits a reading where care is more than a governing principle, or an ethic that frames the rehearsal or performance. Lee's work encourages a care aesthetics approach where those practices of intimacy and care are integral to her work, rather than enablers of it. In the interview with Welton, Lee argues 'the relationship between dance and care is not metaphorical' (2013: 2509) echoing my point above in relation to the balletic game during the *Grandchildren of Hiroshima* rehearsal. It was not care *like a* dance, but here *care is dance is care*: it has in Hatton's words 'a caring aesthetic' (2019: 100). The following from Lee, which is worth quoting at length, is the perfect statement of this non-metaphorical approach:

> In order to dance well and in order to rehearse well, dancers need to have a balance of acceptance of leading and following, of letting go of control, of being in control, or of being just a partner. Just to pick someone up, just to dance with someone you've got to kind of understand how they're feeling

at that moment. There's an ability to connect with people non-verbally and to be empathetic that's really attuned in a dancer, especially in the kind of dance world I'm interested in

(Ibid: 2505).

Later in the interview, Lee follows this close description of 'dancing well' by referring to the 'extraordinary attentiveness' that she 'finds beautiful' (Ibid: 2520). The skill of dancers as they build trusting relations with others, therefore, has a quality that can only be described in terms of its aesthetics. It has an intensity, a heightened quality and a sensation of attention that is itself caring. Here care is necessary for the successful completion of the form, but simultaneously the exquisiteness of the performance is realised in the beauty of that care. Care is not frame, support, or the 'social' distraction worried about by writers such as Claire Bishop, but the action that is completed in the execution of this art practice. Common Dance, therefore, with the diversity of dancers on stage, with many moments of ensemble, dynamic movement, and then moments of intimate near stillness, provides a compelling example of aesthetics of care embedded in both a process and final performance. Of course, as will be developed in the next chapter, writing 'just to pick someone up [...] you've got to understand how they're feeling at that moment' could be a discussion of the skills in nursing care as much as the skills of a dancer. The final point to make here, therefore, is that there is a connection between care in art and the art of care that needs to be deepened.

The perspective on Lee here is echoed in the writing of dance scholar Sara Houston in relation to her analysis of the work of Israeli dancer and choreographer Yasmeen Godder (2020). She argues that 'the structures of reciprocity and exchange' that come from Godder and other similar artists working within practices of community or socially engaged dance, provide 'new ways of imagining dance both as a mode of care for the other and as an evolving choreographic form' (Ibid: 71). Careful art, here, is therefore both a particular mode by which care is realised and an experiment in form. Where this might have started as a social turn as dance artists like Godder move to engage audience members or non-professional dancers in their work, the significance for a care aesthetics standpoint, is that a movement towards the social did not move away from the aesthetic, but also permitted a re-examination of the aesthetics of their practice. The *turn* reanimates rather than diminishes the way they commit to making dance, and the form of dance that is performed. Houston explains how Godder's work, particularly her project *Störung/Hafra'ah*, which was a collaborative German/Israeli initiative working with people who had Parkinson's disease, built on the 'recognition of the need for caring relationships and caring practices when working with individuals different from oneself' (Ibid: 80). She then continues to explain how this has 'elicited new approaches to making dance' (Ibid). The attention to care folds back into a new attention to the aesthetics of her practice. This was not an abandonment of the freedom to take risks in one's artistic practice, constrained by meeting the social needs of participants, but one that in trusting 'the caring structures nurtured through the community sessions and rehearsal process' required Godder to take 'a big risk artistically' (Ibid: 83). As will be discussed later in this chapter, and was touched upon right at the beginning, riskiness is not the artistically bold counter to the timidity of carefulness, but in a world where not taking care is the norm, seeking forms of care-taking provides the greater, and aesthetically more rewarding, risk.

The commitment to what might be called *caring forms* were similarly developed in Godder's work from 2009 called *Stabat Mater,* a performance made of two related pieces, one called *Simple Motion* and the second called at first *Stabat Mater* and later *Simple Action*, which was premiered in a small chapel in Northern Italy. There is an excellent extended analysis of the *performance of care* in these pieces by Sarah Houston (2020), so I do not want to repeat her account here. However, it is worth quoting Houston at length because it illustrates how close relational work between audience members and dancers can develop an intense experience for those participating and a profoundly moving event for those observing. The attention to lifting, weight and balance here echoes the opening vignette where an elder is bathed, suggesting again that we cannot divide one easily as care and one as dance, but need to examine them both for the care aesthetics they enact and demonstrate. They are not *the same* in a simplistic sense, but the context of a domestic bathroom and Italian chapel, cannot be assumed to be the sole determining factors of their aesthetic importance. Houston writes, describing the opening movements in the performance:

> At first in silence, one dancer stands up and walks over to a random audience member. Offering their hand, they talk quietly, inviting them to come into the space with them: 'Hello my name is [...], I would like to offer you, if it's ok, to give me your weight, and slowly we will go down towards the floor. You can really lean on me.' In accepting that offer, the audience member, now participant, falls slowly to the floor in the dancer's arms. Slowly releasing their weight, giving it all to their partner, the participant relinquishes control over their body. Falling slowly, both figures reach the ground, the supporting partner taking care over their charge's head on the marble floor. Once on the floor, the participant is invited to stay there for as long as they want before going back to their seat. Their partner stays for a while too, sitting or kneeling by the other's body [...] The dance work develops by allowing participants to invite other audience members into the space to hold them in their arms and take them down to the floor. There is no obligation to take part. Men hold women, women hold other women, children hold men, men hold men, older and younger bodies fall, keep falling and lying on the ground
>
> *(Ibid: 72).*

The delicacy of the movements here are important, but it is how each one is entirely reliant on a relation with another for it to gain is fluency and grace that is also significant. Echoing the description of relations between participants in the London Bubble game above, the momentary caretaking between two people, has a form and a sensory flow, so that we see the art as careful, and also note that intimate care has a certain artfulness. Again, holding the weight of someone as you lower them to the floor is not a support mechanism that is brought from the background to the foreground as per the analysis of Jackson, but is the centre of the work itself. Care or support are not practices that enable the art to exist, but in these examples of dance, they are the practices by which the form is realised or experienced. Bodies in motion, whether professionally trained or not, seem to require an aesthetic of care both to make that motion possible, but also provide the intensity of experience, an inter-relational beauty, that can be a vital element of these examples of community dance.

One-to-one performance

In the example from Godder above, the intimate lifting and placing that happens between dancer and audience member, if taken in isolation, could belong to the performance form that is known as one-to-one performance (Heddon and Johnson, 2016; Machon, 2017). This is a practice that grew in prevalence and popularity in the early decades of the 21st century, perhaps as an archetype of the shift that was noted at the beginning of this chapter by Lavender as a symptom of a new 'age of engagement' (2016: 21). One-to-one performance is diverse in scope and intent, but linked by its focus on single audience members, whose role might be as active participant in the event, silent witness, or collaborator. While one-to-one performance is a key part of the analysis of *engagement* offered by Lavender, it is important not to assume that it is solely evidence of performance artists commitment to providing experiences of togetherness. Josephine Machon notes a desire for 'non-mainstream audiences' for 'conviviality and congregation' (2017: 23) and argues for this 'politics of connectivity' to be a response to 'the fact that human interaction and ideas around community, caring and compassion are all too absent from our daily lives' (Ibid: 133). While I agree in part with this perspective, and clearly my focus here will be on one-to-one as a caring art form, there is no inevitability to this orientation. Caroline Wake, in her study of the politics of one-to-one performance, illustrates that the modes of participation that it uses 'ranges from the convivial to the confrontational' (2017: 163) and it is important, therefore, to see it is a practice whose commitment to intimacy might not automatically correspond to a practice of carefulness. In some ways, the performance artist focused on here, Adrian Howells, who was one of the most well-known and expert proponents of this form, also shifted along Wake's continuum, where an early work, for example, *The 14 Stations of the Life and History of Adrian Howells* might be deemed more confrontational compared to his later work discussed below. While the desire to *confront* and *shock* audiences is discussed in more detail in the second part of this chapter, the emphasis here will be on how *some* practices of one-to-one performance provide important examples of the interaction between performance and caring.

The work of Adrian Howells is drawn on first to make the case that his work was an example of care aesthetics in practice, but then to make two related points about what an aesthetics of care perspective does for an understanding of it. In the beautiful edition on Howells' work that came out after his death in 2014, Deirdre Heddon and Dominic Johnson present the 'central imperative' driving his work as a 'desire to create intimate, immersive, and transformative encounters with others' (2016: 10). In their words, 'his performances were therefore concerned fundamentally with care, safety, generosity, affirmation, and pleasure' (Ibid). This focus on care and pleasure can be seen acutely in his 2008 performance piece for a single audience-participant *Foot Washing for the Sole*. Machon, in her book on immersive theatres, provides a compelling account of this performance:

> Foot Washing for the Sole [...] is a one-to-one performance that lasts for 30 minutes, always sited in peaceful settings. Whilst washing and massaging the feet with choreographic care, Howells quietly shares thoughts on the symbolic relevance of feet washing, and its spiritual and cultural associations. This allows Howells to reflect on the situation in the Middle East, and on notions of 'peace' and 'service'. All the while he shares these thoughts, Howells completes a careful choreography of washing, drying, anointing and massaging the participant's feet in frankincense oil. As a consequence of the intimacies and philosophies shared, it concludes with Howells requesting permission to kiss the feet
>
> *(2017: 18).*

Here we have an account of a precisely crafted encounter between two people where one attends closely to the other, in a relation that is an act of service. While service can of course slip to servility, here there is a sense of reciprocity as the choreography is negotiated consensually between two people. There is a carefulness running through the relatively short event that is not a permitting structure that allows it to unfold, or the subject matter that the performance is simplistically *about*. Rather an act of care is completed in the planned and delicately executed moments, and that care has an artfulness, or more properly in this account, an aesthetics. Howells' work is not a rumination on care, on its absence in contemporary life, but is an organised experience of care at its sensory best. When interviewed by Johnson about this piece, Howells outlined the precision of the *choreography* highlighted by Machon. He explained 'I painstakingly work out where the soap dish should sit in relation to the essential oils [...] I'm really careful about colours, proximity and the space around things, lighting, temperature, and the way objects and arrangements might be read' (2016: 111). In the language of this book, this is the organisation of a care aesthetic: the minute detailed execution of a caring moment between people constructed through elements of space, human-to-human and human-to-object spatial arrangement, and the attention to the physicality of the relations between participants. Later in the same interview, he elaborates on the precision of this crafting by noting the importance of the different elements of his practice working together. He says, 'it wouldn't matter if I got everything else right if I was asking somebody to put their feet in tepid or cold water' (Ibid). Howells understands this attention to the staging of his work as being an integration between care, the overall impact of the performance and his role as an artist. By failing, in this example by over-looking the temperature of the water, 'it would no longer be caring and kind, and would sabotage the performance, as well as my intention and integrity as an artist' (Ibid: 111).

As with other examples in this section, the claim is that Howells had an expertise, perhaps even a virtuosity, in the aesthetics of care. The attentiveness to the experience of another in *Foot Washing* demonstrates a keen awareness of the complex dynamic of interhuman relations, and how for them to be satisfactory, they need crafting with a sense of what Machon calls the 'multidimensional and holistic capacity of the full human sensorium' (2017: 80). The added emphasis of this analysis, however, is that this is not the same as insisting that artists play a unique role in meeting the lack of conviviality in our daily lives. Yes, Howells helps us understand good care for its sensory, embodied qualities, but my argument is that he points to how interhuman care itself demands an attention to its aesthetics, and at its best, should be a well-honed craft. As before, this is not the Duchamp model, with the artist Howells placing the artefact of care into a 'gallery', or a performing arts festival, thereby designating it as art. Care has an aesthetic already, which is notable in many different settings, and Howells happens to be a highly skilled practitioner of that aesthetic. In a one-to-one performance, in the context of the festival, framing an interpersonal caring encounter as art does, however, enable us to pay close attention to the intimate connection between art and care. Howells makes the case for the aesthetics of the care we share with others to be taken seriously, to be worked at and to be a necessary practice that makes our communal life more liveable.

My second point to draw from the fact of Howells being an exemplary care aesthetician is that he helps us recognise that contemporary accounts of care miss the embodied craft skills needed to make them life sustaining. In terms of the debates on care ethics from Chapter 2, *Foot Washing* appears almost as an extended critique of some of the disembodied accounts that exist in the literature. One direct engagement between Howells and care ethics came in an interdisciplinary research workshop organised in Leeds in the UK, by theatre and performance academic Helen Iball in 2010. This event explored the review process undertaken by Howells to get ethical clearance for the *Foot Washing* performances that were developed when he was a creative fellow at the University of Glasgow. Iball's excellent account of these discussions can be read in the Heddon and Johnson edition (2016: 190–203), where she frames her analysis through the writing of care ethicist Nell Noddings (2013). So, for example, in describing how Howells 'looks at his participant several times, gauging her process, before beginning to wash her second foot', she notes that this 'sequence may be recognised as exemplifying the fundamental components of caring as proposed by Noddings: engrossment, motivational displacement and recognition' (Ibid: 195). Her extended analysis of *Foot Washing* through the framework of care, is a great example of how the literature on care ethics can reveal the dynamics of care that are at play in this, and other, examples of intimate performance. The point that is missing here, however, is how, while Iball is right to read the Howells performance through concepts such as *engrossment*, a performance with an exceptionally well-constructed aesthetic of care in fact speaks back to the care ethics literature. It emphasises that care is practiced and then enacted through bodily engagements. A caring relationship is based on recognition, the 'looking' and 'eye contact' that Iball mentions, but it is also crucially performed through touch, movement, and felt co-presence. It has, in Fintan Walsh's words a 'haptic dramaturgy' (2014: 58). Where writers such as Maurice Hamington animated the care ethics field by drawing attention to the missing body in performances of care (2004), I would argue that Howells' work, so sadly cut short by his death, speaks back to the care ethics field by displaying the vitality and necessity of an aesthetic practice of our care for each other.

Howells will return briefly at the end of this chapter, when in an interview with Dominic Johnson there is a comment about the difference between a high street pedicure and his *Foot Washing* performance (2016: 110). This will be part of the set up for the chapter that follows, allowing me to argue the difference is perhaps a little less clear than we might imagine. For now, we will move to the second part of this chapter, where a series of challenges to careful art will be discussed, either those tendencies that it might be working against, or the opposition that it might face. Clearly many of these have been hinted at in the accounts of practice above. To make the case for the importance of carefulness in art making, they will be spelt out.

Arguments for a careful art

Shannon Jackson has argued that 'whether cast in aesthetic or social terms, freedom and expression are not opposed to obligation and care, but in fact depend on each other' and then comparing her point directly to artistic practice, she notes how 'this is the daily lesson of any theatrical ensemble' (2011: 14). Borrowing from Jackson, the second part of Chapter 3 lays out some of the many *daily lessons* we need to absorb once we accept that free expression and obligated care are mutually dependent. This will include three arguments focused on what the case for careful art is working against, to make the point that certain *obligations* should be welcome to artists and their projects, and neither diminish them nor place unnecessary constraints on practice. Then the implications for this cojoining of carefulness with artistic practices will be examined for how we might develop positive accounts of the way we manage process, relate to audiences and participants, and then can welcome a more integrated, less dichotomous understanding of the relation between artistic practices and everyday life.

In asserting that the aesthetic and the ethical, expression and care in the quotation above, are co-dependent, it becomes clear that placing the artist, and the projects that they create, beyond ethical critique is unsustainable. My first defence of careful art, therefore, is that objecting to art being appreciated for its carefulness because an artist should not be constrained by ethical or in Bishop's words 'pre-established moral criteria' (2012: 238), fails to recognise that artists are always already part of the world, and therefore can rightly be subject to judgement within the various discourses that operate within it. They might have an astounding capacity to present new insight, or re-shape the world in ways that surprise us, but to insist this capacity permits them a pass from critical attention to the ethics of their work, offers them a privilege that is indefensible. Kester points to the tendency 'to endow the artist with the singular capacity for transcendence' which elides their 'situational accountability' (2011: 58) and I agree that this elision is unsupportable. The case for careful art starts with the simple assertion that because art making and artistic projects take place within varied social situations (even a gallery is social context), they have no more right to exceptional treatment than any other category of human practice. Claiming special treatment, insisting that 'the arts' should only be governed by 'properly *artistic decisions*' (Bishop, 2012: 238), has echoes of other dubious claims for exceptionalism. We do not accept priests arguing that their behaviour should only be judged by 'properly theological decisions', or the Masons insisting their practices are only subject to 'properly masonic decisions'. If we accept that care ethics is a reasonable starting point for understanding the way human communities might negotiate more just relations between their members, careful art is no more than a statement that artists and their work are part of, not apart from, these negotiations.

The second argument flows from this first. If the first point was to insist that arts practices no more deserve a special *autonomous* status than any other human activity, the second takes this one stage further, drawing on the discussions from Chapter 2, to insist that autonomy is a conceit that conceals inevitable human interdependence. While some artists historically might have claimed a space for independent action or insisted that they are not beholden to any social constraint, the case for careful art insists that art making relies on a multitude of social contributions, support structures or enabling economic practices, that should be acknowledged rather than denied. On the one hand, this is the plethora of subsidy (for training, venues, and projects) and social support (in education, media, and wider cultural endorsement) but it is also the simpler assertion that art making, even at its most individualistic, relies on human relations for it to be complete. While on the one hand Bourriaud was right, in his seminal work on 'relational aesthetics' (2002), to focus on relations and their importance in contemporary artistic practice, it is an obvious point that *relational aesthetics* more broadly conceived is only an extension of what is evident in many art forms already. Even the most ardent proponent of artistic autonomy would accept a degree of reliance on single or multiple others to engage with or appreciate their practice. Careful art is, of course, both fully accepting of its dependence on others and the world in which it takes place, but also seeks to make a virtue of that interdependence. In being made up of the actions of interdependent humans, whether imbricated in the lives of each other, or embedded into complex institutions or environments, careful art suggests practices that celebrate and examine the forms our inter-reliance takes and the possibilities it contains, should be welcomed. It does not have its creativity, the richness of its aesthetic register, depleted the greater its absorption in its human and material context. In living, collaboratively and carefully within a particular setting, it draws its aesthetic strength from it. This is not a thin form of instrumentalism, or art as a social mirror, but a commitment to developing a dynamic range of aesthetic-ethical practices, nourished the context in which it takes place. In different ways, careful art projects hope to produce protective forms of sociality in an unequal world, and beautiful acts of solidarity in communities that for too long have been brutalised by an insistence that people must survive on their own. Interdependence is, therefore, a source of richness, not a shackle to cast off.

The third assumption that careful art is working against is the sense that success in artistic practice is determined by the degree to which the event or experience shocks, disrupts or forces audiences or participants from their comfort zones. While Kester presents this 'antagonistic relationship' as written into the 'very DNA of modernist art' (2011: 38), it is arguably a DNA that thrives within practitioners and scholars from many traditions as they present what they see as the rightful purpose of artistic practice. This is notably the case in accounts of performances in our *age of engagement* as the treatment of audiences and participants is frequently viewed through the prism of a demand for *confrontation*. Set against this, it might appear that *careful* art advocates a somewhat timid and compliant practice, hardly worthy of a place in the brave world of cutting-edge contemporary art. The starting point of my critique here is the sense that a default of 'riskiness' is a taken for granted objective without consideration of its implications. So, theatre academic Lourdes Orozco simply states that 'risk seen as danger is the core of theatre practice' (2017: 35) and Bree Hadley argues artists need to take their spectators 'out of their comfort zone' if they are to grow and change (2017: 60). Similarly, Bishop asserts that 'unease, discomfort or frustration [...] can be crucial to any work's artistic impact' (2012: 26) where what Jackson refers to as the need to 'disrupt the social' (2011: 14) is the vital signifier of an artist and their art projects' worth. The unquestioned assumption here is that first the people who are attending or participating in these events come from a place of comfort. This is the model, criticised by Kester, of the transcendent artist who has a special insight into the lives of these audience/participants and knows that they need to be shocked out of their complacency. There is an assumption of the peculiar capacity of artists to provide dullard audiences or participants with an affective shove. My argument would be that in the early years of the 21st century this appears to be based on a dubious sociology. Where is this comfort that needs to be dislodged? It is just as likely that people are living lives of discomfort and disturbance and could in fact be longing for a place of comfort. To shock people out of their comfort zones, anticipates a participant whose default life experience starts from ease. Careful art is proposing a movement in the opposite direction, so that artistic practice draws people out of their discomfort zones – perhaps creating a place apart from the daily challenges of economic hardship, mental health struggles, violence, and the many other ills of contemporary society. This might be the exact place in which artistic experiences offer the opportunity for respite and change. The assertion that disturbance leads automatically to positive insight feels a somewhat tired reformulation that suffering is needed for great art. It is perhaps as likely that discomfort leads to dis-ease and diminished lives. This perspective coincides with Jen Harvie's when she admits she is 'wary of prioritizing dissenting art practices' arguing instead that 'pleasurable fun can constructively engage audiences' (2013: 10). In arguing against the automatic dismissal of comfort, the case for careful art suggests that experiences that provide rewarding 'sustenance' (Jackson, 2011: 29), which might in their own way be loud, celebratory, and raucous, should be welcome in a world when disruptive shock is in many ways and for many people already part of everyday life.

The case for discomfort as the driver of artistic ambition, therefore, makes assumptions about the existing life experiences of audiences, spectators, and participants and places artists in an elevated position above them as somehow more knowing and perceptive about the world in whose misdeeds audiences are by implication complicit. Artists are petitioned to 'take risks, to go to extremes, to confront, to challenge, to provoke reaction' (O'Grady, 2017: 12) automatically assuming that challenge and risk operate in a register of confrontation. Careful art, as a proposition, suggests that in a world of disruption and discomfort, the risk might in fact be in an alternative medium of collaborative consolation. There is not, therefore, a binary relationship between the work that on the one hand provokes reaction and takes risk, and work on the other that is comforting and caring. If a 'social art practice seeks to forge social bonds' (Jackson, 2011: 14) it may be an intense, profoundly moving and risk-filled counterpoint to the dislocations and disturbances that exist within a particular community's daily reality. Careful art places the arts practice within communities of participants, and works alongside them, without assuming prior knowledge of the contours of their experiences: without assuming their need for either shock or comfort. It is a proposal for an aesthetics of care, which is a counter to what might be called, slightly tongue-in-cheek, *the aesthetics of scare*. We need to ask who benefits from this fearful aesthetic experience when it might already be part of the fabric of a person's interpersonal daily life and maybe is the last thing they want reinvigorated in an artistic event.

My last point about *the aesthetics of scare* is that when criticising a demand to shock, a comment is being made in both an aesthetic and ethical register. As already noted, Bishop might decry the encroachment of the ethical into the *properly aesthetic*, but the argument of care aesthetics is that this fails to recognise that in many areas of life unravelling the ethical from the aesthetic is far from simple. If we take Bishop's positive account of the Spanish artist Santiago Sierra's 1999 work '250cm line tattooed on 6 paid people', where the artist tattooed a long line across the backs of six Cuban men, we would be mistaken not to comment on the blue-black tattoo scar from both an aesthetic and ethical perspective. The work, repeated on different occasions, for example with four prostitutes in Spain in 2000, 'draws attention to the *economic* systems through which his work is realised' according to Bishop (2012: 223. Italics in the original). This is a form of analysis where suddenly the bodies of the scarred workers become insignificant and merely a form that transfers attention to something else. It misses the aesthetics of the event itself, and the actual tattooed line. Rat Western similarly in her analysis of South African Live Art, argues that we need to avoid 'criticising a participatory work for being undemocractic towards its participants' because 'intentionally disconcerting or discomforting participants' might draw 'attention to such discriminations as they exist in life' (2017: 184–5). Again, the living people involved are artistic material to be manipulated to ends beyond their existence as breathing bodies, and therefore a vital element of the aesthetics of the work is overlooked in the same breath as a complaint about socially orientated arts practices forgetting the aesthetic is made. Although Western argues that anything else would be a 'focus on ethics over aesthetics' (Ibid: 184), in fact on being concerned with discrimination generally (and not as enacted on the bodies of participants) it is her that is focusing on ethics not aesthetic experience. Similarly, Bishop in her analysis is paradoxically concerned more with an *economic system* than an aesthetic one. I would argue that the treatment of participants in an *undemocractic* way is an aesthetic *and* ethical decision: it is potentially *both ugly and unjust*. Hurting someone to make a point about pain, does not suddenly become aesthetically interesting or ethically appropriate because of the quality of the point that that is made. And the tattoo scar in Sierra's work is, from my point of view, ugly in its carelessness and artistry whatever it might *draw attention to*. Careful art is a rejection of the aesthetics of that scar/e.

Dramaturgy of care

Obviously in this brief overview of arguments that place the artist beyond critique, autonomous and happy to disrupt the lives of their audiences and participants, there is a broad stroke commentary being made on many subtle and complex practices that do not necessarily contain all these components or endorse them in a fixed or permanent way. It could also be argued in the shifts towards an 'age of engagement' with different practices of intimacy in performance, the modernist DNA has started to weaken in our collective artistic gene pool. That said these assumptions applied to live art, performance art and certain practices within more participatory theatres and arts practices, do still endure. An important element of a case for careful art is that it is not a demand for a practice that is straightforwardly the opposite to this version of modernist art – a replacement of the confrontational, transcendent, independent artists with his or her intimate, collaborative alter-ego. It is more of an outline of the shape of processes, approaches and experiences taking place over time, in many different artistic practices, some which may be structured as caring practices that take huge risks and are organised in such ways as to disrupt many given assumptions. It is an attempt to delineate an aesthetic-ethic that builds across the life of projects through, in Kester's words, a 'cumulative process of exchange and dialogue' (2011: 12), rather than a narrower attention to momentary or instantaneous shock. The focus on process, and attention to the structures of a process, will be called here a *dramaturgy of care*. This is a term taken from Rebecca Groves and her comparison between the dynamics of caring and the dramaturgy of performance (2017), and then director of the performance group Vertical City, from Toronto, Bruce Barton who reimagines it as a 'dramaturgy of embrace' (2014: 61; 2017: 142). In the proposal for careful art, therefore, the attention is to the dramaturgy by which the care/art is organised. The dramaturgy of care describes the structuring, organising, and unfolding of processes between people and the material of their lives over time.

To call this focus on caring processes a dramaturgy, points to the way care itself is not simply a one-off act that is produced in a singular time-bounded moment. It is, as Groves suggests, composed of 'enduring and relational dynamics that accumulate over time into structures of meaning' (2017: 310). It is therefore multiple moments that are interwoven in the gradual manifestation of relationships, social dynamics, and inter-human bonds. In Groves' work, she uses this understanding of care having a dramaturgy, to offer new insights into the dramaturgy of performance, but here the proposal is that there is an aesthetics in the composition of caring relations themselves, and these might be well-crafted in different health, care, or art contexts. A dramaturgy of care, therefore, might be recognisable in a hospital ward or a youth theatre company. Close awareness of these dramaturgical processes in artistic projects is an alternative to the assumption about the importance of disruption discussed above. Bruce Barton and his collaborator Phil Hansen adopt the *dramaturgy of embrace* as the core principle in their performance work using it as 'an explicit effort to bypass the culture of exploitation and manipulation that characterised so much early twenty-first-century participatory performance' (2017: 143) and similarly Groves sees a shift to notions of ongoing 'continuity and obligation' as a shift from the 'emphasis on sudden disruption that performance theorists typically favor' (2017: 311). This is important for care aesthetics because there is a claim inherent in these arguments that the process, the gradual practice of building and sustaining relationships in a creative practice, has shape or form itself. Thinking through the dramaturgy of care is an exploration of how that form of durational experience is composed.

In many ways Bishop, in objecting to 'today's participatory art' emphasising 'process over definitive image, concept, or object' expresses this dramaturgy when she explains that it 'tends to value what is invisible: a group dynamic, a social situation, a change of energy, a raised consciousness' (2012: 6). Of course, the insistence here, as discussed in Chapter 1 is that visibility is not the only marker of aesthetic experience, and instead those changes of energy, that pulsing of a group dynamic have form: they have a dramaturgy that can be developed and improved. This echoes art theorist Nato Thompson when he argues that 'just as video, painting, and clay are types of forms, people coming together possess forms as well' (2012: 22). The proposition here is that an assembly for the purpose of joint artistic endeavour, whether play making, singing, or preparing a celebratory meal, may not appear as a simple visible object, but it has sensory contours that mean it can be examined for its dramaturgy. The additional claim for a dramaturgy of care is that careful and caring processes of *coming together* are themselves aesthetically richer than those that might miss or fail to attend to the dynamics of the interactions between people and the quality of the relations that develop between them. This is not the same as demanding a 'good group dynamic' between participants to ensure the quality of the artistry of an outcome. Care aesthetics, developed through a well-organised, beautifully composed drama-turgy of care, is inherent in the process itself. Kester writes in his discussion of participatory arts that dialogue itself is 'fundamentally aesthetic' (2011: 13) and I would expand this to say that the full-bodied interactions between groups where they meet, work, and make together is *fundamentally aesthetic*. In many ways this emphasis is borrowing from craft scholars such as David Gauntlett who describes the 'sense of being alive within the process' in a language which validates the importance of the aesthetic experience between people and not as an outcome of the activity (2011: 25). The quality of the experience, for him, comes 'not before or after but *within* the practice of making' (Ibid) and the idea of the dramaturgy of care points to the importance of focusing on the composition of that *within*. Finally, careful art in being experienced through this dramaturgy of care, needs new dramaturgs. These are artist-carers who are skilled in nurturing sensorially rich, careful encounters between people, between people and the materials with which they are working, and between these experiences and the wider world.

There is one additional point to mention about these *new dramaturgs*, before turning to the notion of simultaneity that then anticipates the next chapter. Organising the dramaturgy of care within an arts project demands that the audi-ence, participants, or collaborators are trusted rather than viewed with suspicion. As mentioned above, the tradition of seeking to shock an audience is reorientated to one where participants are welcomed to an experience that might be challeng-ing or risky but starts without assuming a particular state from which they need to be rescued. Clark Baim, psychodramatist and founder of the criminal justice focused company Geese Theatre UK, has developed schemes for theatre-based group work that exercise what for him is a 'duty of care' (2017: 80) and I support his approach but emphasise again that care aesthetics cannot be reduced to the means to secure the ends of good, caring group relations. The practice of exer-cising that duty of care has a sensory quality itself, making it part of and not mere facilitator of the aesthetics of the project. Writers such as Heddon and Johnson (2016: 29) and Machon (2017: 150) have also noted, particularly in reference to the more intimate, immersive, or one-to-one performance projects, that *care for the audience* is a pre-requisite for the engagements that these performance forms seek. This is, therefore, a starting point for a dramaturgy of care that wants to work with audience-participants over time, through a process to the completion of an experience. Trust therefore replaces suspicion as a certain 'gentleness' (Machon, 2017: 150), what a care ethicists like Noddings might call 'engrossment' (2013: 12), is produced across the course of project. A dramaturgy of care needs a dramaturg with a prevailing attitude to audiences, collaborators, participants, or co-artists, who starts from a sense of mutual regard (Hatton calls this 'attunement' (2019: 96)), and then seeks to expand it into dynamic and complex convivial relations as the very substance of the art making itself.

As we move towards chapter four, an examination of artful care, the questions about who these dramaturgs are, who in fact are the artists, and where does this dramaturgy of care take place, start to take greater prominence. Although the writing here has made the case for careful art, and Chapter 4 turns this around to present an account of artful care, as will be clear from the arguments above, ultimately it is the relationship between these two that is at the core of any account of care aesthetics. The final point to make here, therefore, is that the understanding of aesthetics and care, and more broadly the debates between art and society, or Art/Life above in Jackson's words (2011: 29), approach the relationship as one of simultaneity rather than distinction. This means that we are not seeking to make a simplistic aesthetic reading of the social or adding social objectives to practices more traditionally designated art. Rather than a 'slide into sociological discourse' (Bishop, 2012: 17) that forgets the aesthetic, *simultaneity* suggests that we entertain both modes of analysis at the same time because something purely social cannot be disentangled from something purely aesthetic. As Kester notes, we should avoid a 'hygienic attitude on the part of the critic, who must defend art from contamination' (2011: 35) by both accepting the close imbrication of the two and championing the richness of an artistic practice that works with and explores that complex interrelation. The gentle reassurance from Lois Weaver as she speaks to Peggy Shaw from the auditorium has a depth and quality because it presents an ethic of care, but its tone, clarity and context of utterance ensures that it has a sensory, felt resonance in the moment. It both delivers aesthetically and socially, and to see one as undermining the other fails to recognise the remarkable co-existence of both these modes as they were experienced in this performance. At a more intimate level, the touch on a shoulder during the game played in the London Bubble theatre workshop, can only be understood as operating in a simultaneously aesthetic and ethical register. I would argue that this is a straightforward acceptance of the way we would experience this moment. If someone touches another person, you do not split the ethics of that touch (was it consensual, was it welcome, was it violent, was it careful) from its aesthetics (was it rough, was it tender, was it ugly, was it careful). This is not to say that they are the same, but to argue that often they are experienced simultaneously, and to criticise art projects that allow one to be confused with the other fails to recognise how aesthetics is interwoven with 'sociological discourse' in many areas of life. In a chapter by Zoe Zontou on theatre projects with recovering drug users, she quotes the artistic director of Fallen Angels Dance Theatre company, Paul Bayes Kitcher, where he asks, 'does our want to care, hinder the artistic process and the ability of the dancers?' and Zontou concludes that 'safeguarding the participants was prioritised over the aesthetic quality of the piece' (2017: 222). The case for simultaneity would present this differently asking instead how we might locate the aesthetics of the safeguarding and discover means to validate that as part of the quality of the piece. In my brief point about touch above, in the bracketed examples, I placed 'was it careful' in both the ethics and aesthetics parentheses, because ultimately this edition is arguing that, perhaps above other areas, care is a place where ethics and aesthetics are more tightly bound than others.

Simultaneity, therefore, pertains particularly strongly to practices of care. As has been argued across this chapter, art making, particularly in relational, participatory practices, might need care to help it proceed smoothly, and might deal with issues of care in profound ways – but more importantly art making can be an exercise of care itself. This is not care brought to art, but a simultaneous caring through the process of the artistic endeavour. When Anne Basting, in her book *Creative Ageing,* asks the question 'what if care centers really truly became cultural centers?' (2020: 159) she is demonstrating this sense of simultaneity between the two areas of practice. Care centres could become cultural centres, and, for this chapter at least, it is hoped that more cultural centres might understand their roles at care centres.

Michael Balfour, in his work in Australian care homes, makes a similar point to Basting, when he expresses a concern that his account of 'aesthetic caring' is made not to disrespect the extraordinary work of the professionals working in these contexts (2019: 93). As I shift to Chapter 4, my point would be to insist that we need to avoid thinking about the aesthetic caring done by artists on the one hand, and the work of the health care professionals on the other. While there may be differences in intensity or approach, the ambition here is to discover how their work has an aesthetics as well. This is a shift from attention to careful art, to the subject of Chapter 4 which focuses on 'the extraordinary commitment demonstrated by the majority of professionals that work in these contexts' (Ibid) as a practice that has its own aesthetics: as a practice of artful care. This is not to suggest that a focus on the aesthetics of the practices of health care professionals dispenses with the need for the specialist role of artists, but to insist on simultaneity in care aesthetics – that is, understanding it as a register for the sensory, embodied practice of inter-human relations whether it is done by artists, care workers or others. I end the chapter by returning to the work of Adrian Howells, and his intimate performances of tenderness to illustrate this point. In an interview with theatre academic Dominic Johnson, he discussed the staging, preparation, and execution of his work *Foot Washing for the Sole.* Johnson in response suggested the following:

> *There is a qualitative difference between the experience of a one-to-one performance and a commercial interaction – between, say, participating in* Foot Washing for the

Sole *and receiving a high-street pedicure. A key difference, for me, is the aesthetic staging of the situation in your work*

(2016: 110. Italics in the original).

While I would agree with Johnson that there might be a difference in quality between the experience of having your feet washed by Howells and a similar experience in a high-street pedicure, the argument here is that this is not because one has 'aesthetic staging', and the other does not. The approach of care aesthetics is to suggest both operate with an aesthetic register. They both involve the organisation of sensation over time, the arrangement of space, and the execution of touch between people. Where Howells might have the unfolding of tenderness as an objective, and the pedicure might be focused on the treatment of feet or their beautification, they are both involved in the aesthetics of care. One might do this with more heightened skill or singular attention to the dramaturgy of that care than the other, but the point here is to explore how they might be examined more for the similarities than differences. For me, Howells's strength was how he presented an experience that was in dialogue with other experiences of foot care (and tenderness between individuals more broadly), rather than a performance that was dismissive of or inherently distinct from them. Howells had a capacity to stage care beautifully between people and accepting this as an extraordinarily skilful practice of care aesthetics, helps make the demand that other experiences of care, in other contexts of our daily lives, have this sense of quality and depth. Many high-street pedicure salons might, against the odds, be struggling to create aesthetically caring experiences, and with limited economic means, might have success. Howells *careful art* meets the high street's *artful care*, and we need to discover means to point generously to the craft of those foot-washers who do not usually have the attention or limelight. The desire here is to understand how the care aesthetics of artists like Howells and the care aesthetics of workers in pedicure salons might have opportunities to draw from each other.

Chapter 4 takes up this challenge. It does not claim that the work of pedicurists, nurses, homecare workers and many other people in the formal and informal care sectors is inevitably artful or always has the space for the graceful choreographies of care touched upon in this chapter. It does recognise the exploitation and systematic devaluing of people's labour that takes place in many different contexts. But, at the same time, it believes that there are multiple examples of artful care, often in spite of circumstances and resistant to the restrictive demands of under resourced contexts. In performance scholar Kaitlin Murphy's analysis of the performances of care and resistance between women on the US-Mexico border she argues that *resistance is also an assertion of the right to be cared for* (2020: 82) and following her assertion, the resistance here will be the demand of the right of carers to have their capacities valued and celebrated. The purpose of Chapter 4 is, therefore, to explore how valuing and attending to their artfulness might lead to new ways of understanding health and social care, and opportunities for improving the quality of the care that many experience.

4

Artful care

While Chapter 4 is a substantial way through the book, it is important to acknowledge that it was an experience of *artful care* where this project started. My search for a way of understanding care as an aesthetic practice, and for an inclusive approach to thinking about socially engaged arts practices and care practices, did not originate in my position as a theatre practitioner. It started from witnessing the extraordinary care offered to my colleague, Antoine Muvunyi, from the Democratic Republic of the Congo. I understood this health care relationship as an aesthetic encounter, but I was admittedly unsure why I thought it so, and certainly was unclear as to the implications for framing it in this way. There was something of the skill of the physiotherapist in her embodied touch, hold and manipulation of Antoine's fingers and palm. But, also, in the way he responded by holding her in his eyes and expressing to me his trust in the relationship that made the process possible, and bearable. In addition, it did not operate within the standard rules of health institution or clock-based time. Although it did take place in a hospital, it was organised outside the formal constraints of what was a private facility offering its services for free. This allowed for a certain slowness of execution, a theme which will be touched upon below. It was also surrounded with conversation, gentle humour and shared stories. Finally, I knew that throughout the process the physiotherapist was undertaking an additional qualification in hand-based physical rehabilitation, that gave a context for her quality of attention, but similarly suggested that her learning, and her skills, had both a high level of technique and a deep understanding of the nuances of her practice.

The focus of Chapter 4 is how care aesthetics might be applied to health and social care contexts and many of the themes described in the treatment Antoine will be developed in the pages that follow. The practice of health professionals and other carers will be explored for how it might be understood for its aesthetics or for its art (and the difference between the 'art of care' and care aesthetics is

DOI: 10.4324/9781003260066-7

discussed below). This includes accounts from the care literature where the aesthetics of practice is acknowledged, or those that can be understood as belonging to what is called care aesthetics here but might not have used this designation in the original. Madeleine Bunting in her account of the crisis in the contemporary care system in the UK calls care 'that close but poor relation of artistic creativity' (2020: 236) demonstrating that the claim for an artfulness in many care practices is not a new one. As will be discussed below, nursing has been widely discussed for both its art and for what has been called an 'aesthetic pattern of knowing' (Carper, 1978). This is also a reference which goes back to Florence Nightingale and her belief that 'nursing is an art' which 'requires as exclusive a devotion, as hard a preparation, as any painter's or sculptor's work' (1859, quoted in Chinn and Watson, 1994: xv). While the literature on nursing will feature strongly in the pages that follow, it is important to note that the practice of describing a professional practice as an art, is not unique to this profession. For example, social work has been discussed for its artistry (England, 1986) and public health has been criticised for losing sight of 'the art of care' (Hanlon et al, 2012: 3133). The aim of the first part of this chapter is to examine examples from the health and social care literature where either the 'art of care' or aesthetics is discussed, both for the overlap with the argument for an aesthetics of care but also for where the emphasis is different. Examples of practice will be given that operate within the framework of care aesthetics, even if this is not the term used by the writers.

The second part of the chapter examines approaches to the study of care that provide important points of comparison with care aesthetics and the objective is to see how they help enhance the concept or where differences might be important to emphasise. This includes, for example, the notions of bodywork and emotional labour. These then lead to accounts of 'care encounters' or 'moments of care' to illustrate the diversity of care aesthetic practices that are evident in contemporary care services. At the end of the chapter, there will be a brief account of what are called cultures of care, covering relationships beyond the interpersonal such as care environments and the relation between care and time. The ambition of the whole chapter is to draw attention to the aesthetics of care that is at play across numerous health and social care settings, highlighting and giving value to experiences and practices that are too frequently overlooked. Bunting is right to note that care is a relation of artistic creativity, but the starting point here is that its position as *poor relation* needs to be challenged. It is a status that is the result of a gendered division of labour that designates care as 'women's work' resulting in it receiving insufficient critical attention, inadequate levels of investment and limited social and cultural value. Care aesthetics aims to make a modest contribution to demanding that care, despite many struggles faced by those giving and receiving it, is no longer secondary but becomes recognised and valued as a vital, aesthetic practice in itself.

Both Chapters 3 and 4 would fit comfortably within the field of the *health humanities* (see Crawford, Brown and Charise, 2020; Crawford et al, 2015). This research area has documented the intersections between health sciences and multiple disciplines within the arts and humanities. While in terms of the practice-based arts disciplines, this relationship is frequently about what the arts can offer health care, it is also a field that recognises an *art of* health as well as the *arts in* health. Crawford and colleagues mention a traditional approach to the relationship whereby the focus is on 'the potential for arts and humanities to make a real difference to the lived experience of informal carers' (2015: 146). The framework is what the one offers to the other as the assumed point of departure. The shift in this book, and specifically in a chapter called Artful Care, is to one which examines the aesthetics of health care practices, not what the arts as a distinct field might bring to them. This is in fact part of the tradition documented by Crawford, but often articulated as a form of minor key to more familiar preoccupations. So, for example, where there is the suggestion that the performing arts can be understood as health care practices (a concern of the previous chapter) there is also the 'sub-argument that health practices can be understood as ways of being-in-relationship, aesthetically, in time' (Ibid: 86). Similarly, rather than just a 'sub-argument', there is also the assertion in the same edition by Crawford, that the two sides of the *health* and *humanities* relation might be explained under the one rubric where they are both 'relational-aesthetic-temporal phenomena' (Ibid: 89). For *care aesthetics,* this perfectly marks the shift into Chapter 4, where care is understood as a practical activity that has its own aesthetics alongside other arts, and not as a sub domain, or poor relation, of them. The arts and humanities are not in this analysis offering health care a way of understanding itself, or of enhancing its delivery. Instead, there is a parity in that health practices and arts and humanities approaches have a common concern with aesthetics.

The claim that care could be considered an art form, is one that public health researcher Phil Hanlon has explained is not new but suffers from rarely being defined adequately (2012: 2946). The 'art of care', therefore, is a phrase often endorsed but seldom defined with precision. The aim of this chapter is to locate attempts to define what is often seen as an elusive quality in health care practice but also to offer a rationale for why *care aesthetics* might point to a helpful framework for that process of definition. Where the 'art of care' should mean, in the words of nursing educators Peggy Chinn and Maeona Kramer, some property 'essential to the "doing"' of care work itself' (2014: 234), it can frequently take on different and perhaps confusing connotations. While Bunting's assertion of care's poor relation status might be right, the approach of Chapter 4 is to acknowledge the long history of aesthetic debate within health and social care research and as mentioned above, to assert that it deserves greater focus and clarity.

Health and social care scholars' attention to notions of creativity, craft and art is sketched and discussed below. In recent years, this has appeared as a 'cultural turn' in social care research which in many ways parallels the social turn in the arts discussed in the previous chapter. This has been particularly strong in gerontology where an interest in what could be called the aesthetics of the practices of everyday elder care has become influential, and certainly central to the arguments to be laid out here (Twigg and Martin, 2015). The chapter will borrow from 'cultural gerontology', examining practices of 'bodywork' that overlap productively with the account of care aesthetics. This corresponds to the ambition of the chapter to locate artful care within the literature and practices of health and care services themselves. However, practices that are traditionally understood as artistic will be returned to at the end briefly to question the implications for this account for 'non-health professional' arts practitioners. Suffice to say, this is not a repudiation of the arts *in* health and social care, but an attempt to find a different point of departure. This is captured in the questions in Anne Basting's book *Creative Care* (2020), discussed in the previous chapter, where she asks what would happened if we infused 'the creative process into the daily rhythms of care systems' (Ibid: 232) and 'what if we could pour [creativity] into the water of an organization so it spread through its systems to all its staff, the elders, and their families?' (Ibid: 234). There is an integrated approach here, which will echo Basting's vision, aiming to ensure the aesthetics of care, in its positive sense (more below), is encouraged and valued across all practices. So, in Bastings' words when 'home-care workers, Meals on Wheels drivers, and home-visit volunteers, who are so often alone with an elder' feel like they are 'part of a larger, meaningful project' (Ibid: 185) then the distinctions between artful care and careful art might have been fully broken down. They are all participants in the creation of aesthetic experiences with, in this case, elders. The comprehensive approach of Basting anticipates discussion in the books' final chapter about care aesthetics in everyday life, but before getting ahead of myself, I will start with a brief point about 'negative' care aesthetics.

As mentioned in earlier chapters both the words care and aesthetics are used interchangeably for evaluative and descriptive purposes. Care can be inherently positive – *I care for you* – and it can be neutral – *my mother was cared for in a home*. Similarly, aesthetics might assume a positive sense as a synonym for beauty or a purely descriptive designation of a sensory experience that could be positive or negative. I acknowledge that this edition has been seeking out care aesthetic experiences that are positive contributions to the sensorily depleted or cruel practices in diverse settings, but it also acknowledges that practices that are diminished in their sensory register have a care aesthetics but a limited or perhaps unpleasant one. I start here therefore with a brief discussion of negative care aesthetics, what Hilary Moss calls an 'aesthetics of deprivation' (2014: 1032), which is offered as a foil to the positive examples that will follow.

The deprivation described by Moss can be found in the physical environments of health care and the practices located within them. She documents, for example, a hospital setting in which 'everything about the environment was professional, clean, and functional, but the effect was a sterile, clinical environment lacking warmth and humanity' (2020: 430). While environments will be discussed in more detail below, Moss is describing an aesthetic, the result of which was a sense of sterility and coldness. This, according to Moss, is counter to the needs of both staff and patients in these contexts and demonstrated the urgency of seeking out more 'aesthetically pleasing and supportive' ways of organising health care space (2014: 1032). Of course, there is a relation between the environment and the behaviours within it, and an austere context is likely to produce, and be the product of, a set of practices that have a similar quality. It is, therefore, not enough to discuss aesthetic deprivation in terms of the colour of walls, quality of light or other observable features of an external context, it must also be an analytic category for the practical interactions of people. Julia Twigg notes this when talking about the potential failures in care workers' practice. In a choice of words which is emphatically aesthetic, she argues that 'positive cruelty' is perhaps rare, but 'we can imagine rough handling, denigrating language, sneering or nasty words, a silent refusal to recognise the person, the demeaning exposure of the body, cold indifference to embarrassment or anxiety' (2002: 2). *Rough, cold* and *sneering*, are exemplary words for an aesthetic of neglect, or 'negative' care aesthetics. They are clearly not synonymous with beauty or pleasure, but with the sensations, feeling and forms of ugliness that can make care unpleasant and of course abusive.

A critique of negative care aesthetics has been part of the critical work of both practitioners and researchers in health and social care, and it is notable that many of the challenges to the intolerable outcomes of poor care, are presented in a language that might be referred to as a language of aesthetics. For example, professor of nursing, Pam Smith, in the second edition of her pioneering book on the emotional labour of nurses, refers to the experience of a student nurse. This woman was assigned to an elderly care hospital and was 'close to tears because she felt that the old people were being treated like sacks of potatoes – hauled out and in of a bed at the beginning and end of their day with no control over their destiny' (2012: 1). Of course, there is a clear comment on care ethics here, in that the patient is treated as an object and is not able to take any control of the care that they received. However, with the bodily practice, the roughness of the handling, being commented upon, I would argue this is also an aesthetic argument. The craft, the style of the embodied practices of the carers, lacked precision, warmth, and had limited focus on the needs of the person to whom it should have been directed. The aesthetic experience – *like a sack of potatoes* – was cruel and perfunctory. As Chinn and Kramer note, drawing this language directly into the idea of negative aesthetics, a 'blunt aggressive style is aesthetically uncaring' (2014: 254). The broader case here is that histories of systemic underfunding of care services have shaped that style so that widespread economic and social neglect has installed an aesthetics that is itself austere.

In contrast to the roughness and ugliness of poor care, there are numerous examples of *positive* care aesthetics documented in the social care literature. The argument for care aesthetics is designed to be a critical one, and therefore it is right to point to those instances when the care is wanting, and use the aesthetics register to question practices of limited bodily and sensory quality. However, the emphasis in the next section will be on examples where a positive care aesthetics can be pointed to as a way of outlining what an enriched experience might be, rather than what it is not. Five examples are offered, and the source will be quoted at length in each case. The aim is to examine different settings connected to health and social care (here they are an outpatient clinic, several hospitals, a dementia ward, and a care home hair salon) to hear a variety of voices but also to note some of the features that connect across the examples they present. This is not a comprehensive selection but intends to give a flavour of care aesthetics from the perspective of health and social care commentators, and to be illustrative of many of the themes which will then be considered in the remaining parts of the chapter. All five quotations will be given consecutively, and patterns that repeat across them will be discussed below.

British author and musician Marian Coutts wrote an award-winning memoir about her husband's illness and eventual death called '*The Iceberg*' (2014) that is discussed by Bunting in her book '*Labours of Love*'. In her interview with Coutts, she quotes her as follows:

> When Tom was in hospital, I was aware of the charismatic power he had, even when he had no words. Once, I arrived early at the hospital to give him his clothes. The curtains were round his bed and three women were giving him a bed bath; they were talking in several languages. It was an amazing image to stumble on. Tom was totally relaxed. It was like a private party. I couldn't have arranged it better. I certainly couldn't have bought it. It was priceless. It was important, I felt, to bear witness to that kind of work, which is low paid and undervalued. It needs to be spoken about [...] You could feel the levels of attentiveness in staff from the way they walked, their tone of voice, their touch. One consultant was under huge pressure, but she managed to keep that hidden from us. She made us feel like she had all the time in the world for us – to manage that professionally and personally is high art. It was gobsmacking
>
> *(2020: 201).*

From Chinn and Kramer describing the work of a nurse in an outpatient clinic:

> Presley works in the orthopedic (sic) clinic of a large urban hospital and uses aesthetic knowing with each young child who comes for cast removal. It is aesthetic knowing that helps him remove the cast in the least distressing way for the child. Presley understands that this child likely sees a large person approaching her leg with an electric cutter and other tools that resemble those in her father's woodworking shop. Presley might use a combination of distraction and humor as well as careful timing to move through the required procedure in an artful way
>
> *(2014: 33).*

From Smith in her analysis of the emotional labour of nurses:

> it was the way the staff responded to her faither's rapidly changing condition, making themselves available during such a difficult, unpredictable

and emotional time. Although the ward was a short stay medical assessment unit with a fast patient throughput she found this did not detract
from a ward ethos that was "so helpful from the top down". Sister Ronda
described one particular staff nurse whose knowledge of pain control and
recognition of "the little things" ensured Mr Ronda's comfort, as well as
supporting her to be with him as he lay dying and when he died. It later
turned out that this staff nurse had been through such a traumatic experience when her own parent died, and she was determined to ensure patients
and families should only receive the very best end-of-life care possible.
And she was able to do this because the senior sister was always there in the
background promoting an ethos of care

(2012: 202).

From Caroline Swarbick, John Keady, and Elizabeth Sampson in their account of
a researcher moving from non-participant observation to participant observer in
her encounter with a distressed elderly patient who died soon after this account:

I walk around the bed to the empty chair and pull it forwards and towards
the bed so that Amy can see me and we make eye contact. I introduce
myself by my first name and ask if she minds me sitting with her. She smiles
at me. Amy immediately starts to shout loudly for "Alice". I calmly ask
who Alice is and she shouts "Mam, Mam". Amy starts crying and instinc-
tively I reach out and stroke her hair and hold her hand, which she grips
tightly. Amy stops crying and looks directly into my eyes. I ask her if she
minds me stroking her hair, to which she replies "it's lovely". I carry on
and Amy continues to shout for "Alice", whilst looking towards the corridor at the end of the bay. Suddenly, she stops, turns her head to me and says
very matter-of-factly: "they tried to cut him out, but he wouldn't open his
eyes" [...] She then starts to scream very loudly, shouting "Mam, Mam" at
the top of her voice. Her gaze darts around the room in a distressed manner. In a calm and soft voice, I continue to reassure Amy predominantly
through physical touch, of which she is responsive. I am not sure how
much she is aware of my presence. I stroke her hands and face. Amy looks
at me and smiles

(2017: 204).

From Richard Ward, Keady, and Campbell's study of hair care in an elderly care
home salon:

Slow-motion video-analysis also helped to reveal the intricate nature of
sink work. Thermal, haptic and multi-sensory experience is interlaced
with apprehension and anxiety for many clients while the hairdresser com-
bines touch and talk both to reassure and distract. Some clients were asked
to count to ten, others strategically engaged in animated conversation and

by taking advantage of her physical contact with clients the hairdresser could offer a reassuring back rub or accentuate the slow massaging of their scalp

(2016a: 1293).

One of the first things to note across these examples is that the phrases aesthetic knowing, fine art and art are used. The language of the arts is explicit, not in every example, but its use does illustrate immediately that the argument for care aesthetics, shortened to artful care here, is not something that comes to these practices from outside but is frequently articulated by those experiencing them. The concept of aesthetic knowing, originating in the work of nursing scholar Barbara Carper (1978), is vital for understanding how aesthetics and art have been discussed in relation to nursing practice, and it is discussed in more detail in the next section. There are differences between the art of nursing, or art of care, and the idea care aesthetics that are significant and will be discussed below. Besides these explicit art-related comments, each of the examples indicate a focus on the patient or client, a quality of attention and also a sense of an engagement with a well-tuned insight to meet their different needs. The skills used to do this include touch and different ways of speaking, expressed in terms such as 'tone of voice' or humour. These encounters are explained as multi-sensory, combining handling, speaking, and crucially timing to ensure a considered process which creates a certain impression or ethos that is experienced bodily. Some of the interactions here are interpersonal, a relationship between a carer and a cared for, but some are concerned with more complex relational combinations, including those witnessing care, or relying on care for one of their loved ones.

While each of these quotations demonstrate an appreciation of the aesthetics of care, in its enriching, positive sense, they also express a sense of surprise that this quality of engagement is possible. There is an implicit awareness that normally constrained work schedules and demanding individual timetables seem to dissolve or even are jettisoned to ensure a practice that is truly attentive and appropriately caring of the patient. Often care aesthetics is therefore found in implicitly countercultural practices done *in spite of* expectations of time-bound or less sensorily engaged practices. A beautifully executed aesthetic of care, therefore, benefits from a sense of presence, its own expanded notion of time, a range of sensory and embodied skills, a close connection with and attunement to another, and occasionally a suspension of certain practice norms. As explained above, these examples are not representative but merely illustrative of an aesthetic register in accounts of health and social care, that demonstrate that care aesthetics belongs to this field in its own right. The remainder of this chapter aims to explore the themes that emerge from these accounts in greater detail, situating them in a literature on nursing, health, and social care. The final part of the chapter deals with specific practices, such as touch, and this draws on existing traditions in nursing scholarship, exploring the aesthetic 'pattern of knowing' in particular.

Barbara Carper wrote her seminal article 'Fundamental patterns of knowing in nursing' in 1978 and it has produced substantial debate across nursing scholarship and nursing practice since then. Its basic premise was that the knowledge that nurses drew on in their practice included four main patterns of knowing. These were *empirics*, that is scientific understanding, *ethics* as the moral grounding of knowledge, *personal knowledge* of the self and others and finally *aesthetics* or the art of nursing. Peggy Chinn and Maeona Kramer have added a fifth pattern, they call 'emancipatory knowing' (2014: 26) which designates the understanding that encourages nurses to pursue changes in the structures and practices that create inequalities or poor treatments in the first place. While the intention of delineating the patterns was to name the different resources that a nurse might draw on to develop her or his practice in a holistic way, of course in creating different categories there is also a possibility that they would be compared or set in opposition to each other. This is most acute in the tendency to set aesthetic knowing against empiric knowing, so that technical and scientific skills of nurses are positioned as the natural opposite of aesthetic based skills, and of higher value in the broader hierarchies of power in different health care systems.

While Gosia Brykczynska, in her work on nursing 'wisdom', has noted that 'of all the aspects of nursing, the artistic and aesthetic ones are the least commented and understood' (1997: 45), in fact there has been extensive commentary on the concept of aesthetic knowing and the 'art of care' (for example, Chinn and Watson, 1994; Contreras Ibacache, 2013; Rovithis, 2002; Siles-González and Solano-Ruiz, 2016; Wainwright, 2000). Some of this work has sought to centre nursing studies and training within Carper's patterns of knowing (notably the work of Chinn and colleagues) and others have attempted to question its continued purchase, suggesting instead a move away from the boundaries it creates (notable in the work of Julie Duff Cloutier and colleagues, 2007). The argument here will start from Carper, to explore the definition of 'aesthetic knowing' and its corollary the 'art of nursing' and then suggest some of the problems that emerge from both that definition and the extensive debates prompted by Carper's original work.

The first point to note about the aesthetic pattern of knowing is that it is used as a phrase almost interchangeably with 'the art' of nursing. Art and aesthetics are thus somewhat indistinguishable so for example Chinn and Watson refer to the 'art and aesthetics of caring and healing' (1994: xiii) without automatically differentiating them or noting whether the use of art signifies a nurse's practice as an art or if it is 'art-like'. The skill of nursing might be 'like an artist's brush' according to Karen Breunig in her account of how the absorption of an artist in their work is comparable to the feeling of absorption in a nurse-patient relation (1994: 201), but again it is unclear if 'the opportunity to be an artist' (Ibid) is the same as actually being one. Chinn and Watson in the following definition of the 'art of nursing' suggest the differences between art and aesthetic in a way that develops the distinction to be made here. For them:

> The art of nursing [...] includes intentional auditory, visual, sensory, olfactory, and tactile art or acts [...] Among these are purposive movement, touch, sound, color, form, nature, and so on. Nursing as art is lived, expressed, and cocreated in the caring moment [...] the aesthetic character of the expressive form of caring, as revealed in the perception and action of the nurse, includes direction, force, balance, and rhythm
>
> *(1994: xvi).*

The description here links back to the examples above that demonstrated the importance of multiple sensory practices. However, it is the phrase 'aesthetic character of the expressive form of caring' that is crucial because it asserts that caring as a form has an aesthetics, a proposition which is central to the argument of this chapter. There is a problem, however, in that this is revealed in the perception and action of the nurse rather than as is suggested in the previous line as something cocreated in a caring moment. Rather than these two terms – art and aesthetics – being interchangeable, therefore, I want to insist on a distinction between them, linked to the notion of a co-created caring moment. The art of care will be used here as the activity of the nurse, an artistry of the person caring, located in his or her capacity realised in a moment. Aesthetics, on the other hand, is about the form and feel of that moment as it is experienced between all those present. The first distinction to make, therefore, from Carper's notion of an aesthetic pattern of nursing, and the adoption of the art of nursing as its metonym, is that by starting from a knowing of a single person, there is a danger that the focus becomes about individual capacity rather than the shape of a moment created in the relation between at least two people. Contreras Ibacache repeats this when, in his work exploring the evidence for an art of nursing, he defines it as a nurse's 'use of his or her internal creative resources to transform the experience of patients and co-workers' (2013: 333). Care aesthetics is used to avoid this focus on the individual and instead aims to examine the sensory and embodied experience of care between people. This, of course, might be instigated by the craft-like skills of a health care practitioner, but is as likely to be an experience that emerges from the awareness and response of a patient, the interrelated actions of multiple care workers, perhaps the family members visiting, and then the dynamics of a physical environment that shapes and prompts certain feelings, movements and rhythms of engagement. When Mel Gray and Stephen Webb write about the history of social work being discussed as an art, in a parallel account to those that debate nursing, they complain 'the worker's talents are typically lumped together into something called "the art" of practice, but without clear definition about the meaning of the term' (2008: 183). I agree that the definition does need greater clarity but would add that the problem comes from starting from the 'worker's talents' and not how their real time practice with the people in which they are in relation produces dynamic aesthetic experiences in which multiple factors play a role.

Having a greater clarity about the difference between the art and the aesthetics of nursing, therefore indicates why care aesthetics is proposed as something distinct from the art of care. While this chapter does use the term artful care as a shorthand point of comparison to the previous chapter's careful art, my focus is on the sensory shape and feel of a caring encounter, and not only the particular skills of one contributor. That said drawing attention to the skills of the carer does help illuminate important contributing factors to care experiences. The positive element of Carper's framework is that it has enabled both a focus on certain aspects of a health professional's work and in turn given it a value that is often elided. When Smith notes a problem with a division between 'empirics' and 'aesthetics' by explaining how the more senior nurse does 'the "tricky dressings" and complicated medicines' where the untrained carers on the other hand just make 'people happy' (2012: 20), her argument is that 'just' to make people happy is a combination of a set of complex 'caring gestures' that should be recognised. The hierarchy between the 'scientific' work and the 'softer' interpersonal should be challenged. While it is clear many health care settings have seen a gradual marginalisation and devaluing of the sensory skills of staff and a delegation of the more tactile and embodied practices to the lower paid, the emphasis here is that there should be no diminutive, no 'just', in the way these capacities are discussed or recognised. Caring gestures, in all their diversity and context-sensitive complexity, need attention and a commitment to their flourishing, as a way of opposing these hierarchies and countering some of the austerities that accompany them. 'Making people happy' is a vital part of nursing and many other caring practices. Of course, even as we mention how they have often been separated from the more highly valued technical skills in nursing, Carper's differentiation of 'scientific' and 'aesthetic' patterns of nursing and the distinction it seems to delineate, needs to be challenged by insisting that in fact they are often interwoven parts of the same practice. While warm words to a struggling patient might exist in a different register to fitting a canula, the argument here is that each have a technique, and there is a sensory, crafted element of both, and importantly they might co-exist as part of the successful completion of a single procedure. At best, there is an aesthetic knowing in the technical and a technical knowing in the aesthetic.

The focus in the 'art of care' literature on the skills of the health care practitioner, has also led to a language that suggests there is a something of an elusive nature to the practice. *Aesthetic* becomes not a descriptor of an experience brought about by identifiable actions, but a signifier of a practice based upon almost mysterious and inexpressible intuition. Cloutier and colleagues have been particularly critical of this tendency as a response to the work of Carper, seeing her designation of empirics as that which is generalisable, and describable, and the aesthetic as 'beyond articulation' (Duff Cloutier, Duncan and Hill Bailey, 2007: 2) as an unfortunate starting point, creating an unhelpful divide. They argue against *aesthetic* becoming a synonym for the ineffable in nursing practice and insist instead that this trend is more an indication of the immaturity of qualitative enquiry, a feature of the time that Carper wrote her original article, than an accurate description of divisions in nursing practice. So rather than frame an aspect of caring practices as 'difficult to understand' (Chinn and Kramer, 2014: 227) or suffering from the dilemma that 'you know when you act artfully [but] you can never fully explain what you did' (Ibid: 236), the argument here, in agreement with Cloutier, is that we should be finding a language and methodology for capturing this enduring part of health care practice, rather giving it an analysis pass because it is 'art' and therefore unexplainable. This is not to deny the care experience as a situation-dependent moment that has particular rather than universal attributes, as discussed in Chapter 2. Rather it seeks to meet the challenge of identifying the elements that are brought to a meaningful and 'positive' care aesthetic moment. In many ways, writers such as Chinn and Kramer who suggest the unobtainable or unrepresentable nature of the aesthetic knowing pattern of nurses' practice are also those who do articulate behaviours that are likely to craft powerful caring experiences. When they note that it is a practice 'expressed through the actions, bearing, conduct, attitudes, narrative, and interactions of the nurse in relation to others' (2014: 33), they demonstrate that there are ways of explaining those capacities that make up this particular practice. The challenge is to improve and expand the discursive register rather than rely on formulations that seem to endorse the 'art of nursing' as a quasi-mystical endeavour. Aesthetic experiences need a language, a way of capturing how they flow across time, and this makes Carper's patterns useful in starting an exploration of those aspects of practice. However, the different patterns, empirical, ethical, personal, and aesthetic, should be used in an integrative way to start describing and valuing the dynamics of nursing, where the aesthetic component is understood as a living part of their complete skill set rather than a particular term for all those parts of a nursing that cannot be understood under the other forms of knowing. Of course, the implication is that they are also equally important for other health care professionals and care workers, and the integration of 'aesthetics knowing' across care practices should not be one delegated only to the lowest paid.

The discourse of the 'art of care' being the zone of practice beyond categorisation or beyond description, produces two additional confusions about the use of the word 'art' which have implications for the discussion of care aesthetics. The first is that commentators who might assert that 'no one, through pen or canvas, will ever be able to entirely capture the true art and the caring spirit of nursing' (Chinn and Watson, 1994: xiv), also argue that this inexpressible nature can be represented 'symbolically [...] as actions, sounds, or pictures, or in metaphoric language such as poetry or story' (Ibid: 24). The art of nursing, therefore, which is beyond our ability to express it in ways that might be more familiar to the social sciences, leads to the necessity of an artistic treatment of that art form. Waraporn Kongsuwan repeats this in her suggestion that 'aesthetics in nursing' is 'revealed through artistic expressions' (2020: 768). Here we have an *art of* the art of nursing which shifts attention from the aesthetics of the care moment, to a focus on attempts to portray that moment in a range of different expressive

forms. Of course, this is not to deny that poetry, visual art, or theatre which deals
with caring practices is of no value. The suggestion is that this demand for artistic
representations of care practices confuses further the expression 'art of care'. It
means there is problematic lack of clarity as to whether the 'art of nursing' is a
term referring to art of the care experience itself, or artistic work which is made
in response to the practice of care. The purpose here is not to disparage the artistic renditions or explorations of care, and in fact they might be excellent ways of
processing the care that is experienced. However, for care aesthetics the 'art of
care' does not need an art of 'the art of care' to make it have value or meaning
as an aesthetic practice. Care aesthetics insists that care has an aesthetics in itself
and an exploration of a care moment, and the skills enacted in its realisation, are
worthy of detailed attention.

If accounts of the 'art of care' discuss artistic representations in a way that
takes our attention from the caring moment to make the 'art made from care' a
focus of analysis, there is a secondary problematic outcome. It leads to a tendency
in training programmes whereby developing aesthetic knowing can focus on
artistic practices outside the care moment, encouraging students to represent care
in different art forms, and then critique these representations, as a surrogate for
developing their 'artful care' practice. While there is no problem with students
taking health professional qualifications being taught fine art or poetry as part of
their courses, it is a confused notion of the 'art of care' or 'aesthetic knowing' that
makes this the process by which they learn to bring a sense of well-honed skill to
the caring encounter. Judging the short story or poem a nurse writes about her or
his work experience as an attempt to assess their art of care, draws attention away
from care itself as an aesthetic practice. Care needs to be artful, to create rich
aesthetic experiences that are life sustaining for those involved, and this needs
the practice to be considered in its own right. We do not automatically learn
poetry to be better at painting or learn to paint to improve the quality of our
dance. Care involves an elegance and precision of touch, a deep understanding of
presence, an awareness of body movement and a responsive verbal and embodied
relational understanding of others and the space in which they inhabit. These are
capacities, skills and ultimately virtuosities that someone brings to a moment that
are realisable by focusing on them and do not need alternative art forms to take
their place. Of course, a care practitioner who develops a certain sensibility to
others and their environment through an experience of other arts forms, might
become a more sensorily aware human being, who may in turn be able to transfer
their sensibility to the crafting of moments of care. However, the argument here
is that the art of care – to shift from its poor relation status – need not defer to
other arts to make it valuable or successful.

In the argument up to this point there are a set of capacities of a carer which
are embodied, sensory, involve the voice and movement, an awareness of the
other and one's position in space. The development of these as an interrelated
set of well-honed and flexibly enacted behaviours can be called the art or craft
of care. For the purpose of the discussion here the distinction made between art

and craft is deliberately left unresolved. As was seen in Chapter 1, where craft was used for the skill of Shoji Hamada, the physiotherapist and the axe maker, the aim is to disturb the hierarchy between the activities of artists and craftspeople so that both can be considered for the finely developed skills used in the execution of their practice, and an integrated sense of its beauty and capacity for stimulating a heightened degree of sensory experience. The significance here is that the craft of care focuses on the capacities of one unit in the care experience, and not the contours of the whole. The remainder of the chapter will be dealing with a series of discussion points where this relation is played out, so that the caring encounter becomes the focus of attention, even though as will be shown below, discussions of care practices still orientate themselves more to the producer not receiver of that care. While much of the literature focuses only on what the carer contributes, making a case for care aesthetics means giving proper attention to how a care moment can be reciprocal and determined by the actions and responses of multiple people, and multiple factors.

The shift from skills input focused – the art of care – to attention to the sensory experience of care – care aesthetics – is demonstrated in nursing scholar Fredriksson Lennart's work on caring conversations. At first his analysis offers an excellent account of the 'aesthetic knowing', in Carper's language, of the nurse who must exhibit a sense of 'being there' with the patient. This involves:

> Physically attending behaviour, sensitivity to body language, use of touch in a judicious way to comfort or express concern, making eye contact and leaning forward toward the other. Listening, comfortable silence, and communication of understanding of the patient's experience
>
> *(1999: 1170).*

However, a heightened capacity is then noted when the nurse is able to demonstrate not just being there, but 'being with' the other. At that moment there is a 'flow of feelings between two persons with different modes of being in a shared situation, in which the one caring is touched by the patient's feelings' (Ibid). It is this *being with* in care that care aesthetics is seeking to name and develop. It corresponds directly to the approach taken by Mel Gray and Stephen Webb in their discussion of the *art of social work*, where they are seeking to make the distinction between a focus on the virtuosity of the social worker and the more collective understand of the aesthetics of a co-created moment. The 'art' in their words 'is immanent in the mutuality of the caring relationship and not merely in the qualities of the individuals doing the caring or being cared for' (2008: 183). It is not the 'interior aesthetic process of individual creativity' (Ibid: 191) but a 'myriad of factors' such as 'the client–worker relationship, professional requirements, agency environment, social policy and so on' (Ibid: 183). This is precisely the differentiation that care aesthetics is seeking to make. It shifts attention to what Julia Twigg, in her account of bathing elders, refers to as 'the dynamics of the care encounter' where 'production and consumption collapse into one another' (2002: 1).

The next sections of the chapter will move away from those parts of the health care literature that use terms taken from art or aesthetics, to explore other frameworks which relate to and are usefully compared to care aesthetics. Each one is important in its own right, and will be explored for how an aesthetic perspective might challenge the ways they are discussed. They will then be used to illustrate, following Twigg, where they do and where they do not demonstrate a collapse between production and consumption, so that it is the complexities of the mutually experienced moment that become the focus. The first area will be *bodywork*, and its important subsidiary *touch*, before moving onto the link between bodywork and the broader field of emotional or affective labour.

Bodywork

To create a care aesthetic experience there is often 'bodywork' that takes place between the different participants. According to Twigg this is a social or health care activity that 'involves working directly on the bodies of others' with an intention that ranges across the 'medical, therapeutic, pleasurable, aesthetic, erotic, hygienic, symbolic' (2002: 137). Bodywork has gained attention in explorations of care and health as a way of acknowledging an area of practice that is too frequently overlooked. In some ways, the hierarchies of health care mean that progress is measured in the movement a staff member makes away from their direct contact with the bodies of patients. There is a perception that one's status shifts from 'dirty work on bodies to clean work on machines' (Ibid: 138) and therefore the focus on bodywork aims to draw attention to a less frequently documented area of practice, and also insist that it has a level of skill and complexity in execution that deserves recognition. While a care aesthetic moment might not involve a physical interaction between bodies, the suggestion here is that bodywork is a helpful starting point in recognising the embodied practices that a person might bring to an encounter. Frequently the aesthetics of care is heightened through the bodily interactions that happen across the experience. It is significant in the quotation from Twigg above that she mentions medical and aesthetic practices under the auspices of her definition of 'bodywork' and for the argument here this should mean that we examine the body practices of the nurse alongside the beautician as related categories of analysis. Bodywork is a useful term because it has the effect of drawing attention to the form, intention and feelings associated with intimate practices, and simultaneously, how through bodily contact some of the boundaries between different bodywork practitioners might be tested. Twigg lists 'doctors, nurses, careworkers, alternative practitioners, hairdressers, beauticians, masseurs, sex workers, undertakers' as those involved in bodywork (Ibid: 137) indicating a category of labour that cuts across numerous groups. While on the one hand these distinctions are important to document, thinking about care aesthetics in the context of bodywork throws light on the points of connection, and asks how caring and aesthetic experiences might be woven together within the same practice. The act of working with the body of another – bathing, cleaning, holding – while belonging to different contexts, and with different objectives in the moment of execution also cannot be disaggregated neatly into therapeutic or pleasurable, symbolic or medical. Of course, touching a shoulder to prepare a vaccination and touching a shoulder in a massage are qualitatively and practically different actions. The argument here is that by drawing them together under the category of bodywork, and adding an attention to aesthetic experience, we can also note how they have complex resonances of felt response that might overlap and invite comparisons.

Of course, bodywork is not a co-equivalent concept with care, or care aesthetics. Writers such as Twigg (2002) seek to make a distinction between formal care work, body labour, as distinct from more informal bodywork. While I agree that the structures and procedures, and ultimately contracts and regulatory frameworks, that govern labour on the body, make it difficult to compare to body practices that take place informally, perhaps in the family or amongst acquaintances, the slight difference in emphasis here is that the affective *similarities* in experiences involving embodied care across different areas of life are important to point out. Holding your partner's hand and holding the hand of a patient are distinct practices, but care aesthetics seeks to comprehend the joint contours of feeling that structure these encounters and acknowledge how they compare. Bodywork might be holding someone's hand, but the word *work* sometimes obscures the aesthetics of an experience, designating it *mere* task. Of course, it can be hard work, laborious, but to understand it fully we need to explore how an experience draws on embodied practices of care across multiple settings and how it might have qualities that blur the boundaries between different contexts. While bodywork as a concept helps focus attention on those who have direct contact with the bodies of others, it is useful to hold onto a broader category of 'body practices' so that we can understand how bodily care across settings draws on skills, feelings and techniques that exist in both professional and more informal settings. The parent who undertakes the body care of their child creates an experience of that moment that will differ from the nurse in a hospital ward who is required to execute the same care for their young patient. However, to understand the shape and feel of care aesthetics, we must examine the embodied practices across both moments that might have similarities and borrow from each other. The politics of care aesthetics and bodywork, both their problems and possibilities, are often embedded in these comparisons, and how boundaries are crossed, willingly and unwillingly, between the informal and formal, the domestic and the public.

Touch

The action by which a great proportion of bodywork, or body practices, is executed is through touch. An examination of the role of touch in care illustrates how opening different practices to comparison and not erecting barriers between them is helpful. The role of touch in care, and its place in care aesthetics, demands attention, therefore, so that practices from a variety of contexts can be examined for how they differ and yet also borrow from each other. Focusing on care aesthetics does not say that the touch of a homecare worker on the arm of an elderly person is the same as the touch from their adult child as they comfort them. It is arguing that we need to allow these two activities to be brought alongside each other to note how they create or do not create similar patterns of experience, rather than insisting on them being distinct social processes that need to be dealt with under different forms of analysis. Following on from this, touch is also important for its inherent reciprocity. This is in the broad sense in how, in Eve Kosofsky Sedgwick's words, 'the sense of touch makes a nonsense out of any dualistic understanding of agency and passivity' (2003: 14) but also practically in how touch can be 'valuable process' that 'benefits both the service user and the care provider' (Elliot-Graves, 2021: 76). One limiting factor in discussing bodywork in care is that it focuses predominantly on the practice of the carer. As discussed above, this is a focus on the art of care, rather than care aesthetics, because it places an emphasis on the craft of one person brought to the care experience. Bodywork as a concept is helpful for bringing an area of activity that Twigg is right to call a 'zone of silence' (2002: 141) to attention. However, we need to ensure it does not mean we overlook the *work* of the body of the person who is being cared for. Touch in being experienced inter-corporeally, is a vital site of analysis to focus on this mutuality at the heart of a care experience.

In her book on the politics of touch, drawing on the phenomenological work on Merleau-Ponty, Erin Manning focuses the 'aesthetics of moving bodies' that are processual (2007: 60). Touch for her is emblematic of her assertion that senses are not 'given to another or withheld' but part of a process that invents worlds between people (Ibid: 92). The relationship made through touch is one that involves both the person reaching to another, and their touch back (Ibid). Here we do not have bodywork by the carer with the body of a client, but a body practice that is in fact completed by two people in a moment of connection. Of course, this might be more than a dyad, involving multiple actors in a network of connections, but the point to emphasise is that touch can be understood as the moment of an aesthetic experience that, as discussed in Chapter 1, occurs *between* people. It is in Kosofsky Sedgwick's words potentially a moment of 'haptic absorption' (2003: 22). Again, this is exemplary for the argument of this chapter as it seeks to point to the difference between concepts such as 'art of care' and care aesthetics, and here bodywork and care aesthetics. While artists have a craft, a deftness in their touch, care aesthetics in drawing on care ethics, seeks to point to its responsiveness and sense of being completed with another. The account above of the researcher touching the hair of the elderly patient is a form of, in Constance Classen's words, 'tactile aesthetics' (2020: 74) because it was 'lovely' for the women but also because the act produced a sensory experience in the researcher 'stroking her hair'. While the article by Swarbick and colleagues does draw attention to the boundary challenging touch of the researcher, clearly the moment described was significant for the powerful affective sensation of a relationship created between the two people. Care aesthetics, by noting the craft of touch, is proposing closer scrutiny of the experience that emerges in the co-touching that happens in multiple care relationships and the pleasures and discomforts that might exist for those involved. In turn it focuses on the broader contribution of touch to developing what Luke Tanner calls, in his analysis of contemporary dementia care, 'enriched caregiving environments' in places where it is too often denied (2017: 187).

There are two additional points to discuss about touch and care aesthetics in this context. The first is related to how touch is divided into distinct categories. So, for example, Mark Paterson, in his work on therapeutic touch, explains that there is 'task-orientated' and 'expressive' touch (2006: 2). Similarly, Kathleen McCann, in her analysis of the way nurses touch their elderly patients, discusses 'procedural or instrumental' and then 'expressive or affective' forms of touch (1993: 839). These categorisations are expressed in comparable language by Chinn and Watson as a 'central element in the expression of nursing's art/act' (1994: 36). For them how 'artistic touch is distinguished from technical touch' is not fully understood but 'nurse artists, without doubt, are making such a distinction' (Ibid). The argument here, however, is that this distinction is overstated and perhaps presenting touch as a practice with multiple functions nested within each other is more accurate. If a nurse puts her or his hands around the shoulders of a patient to enable a walk down a corridor, this is simultaneously a technically supportive and an expressive act of touch. Returning to the aesthetics outlined in Chapter 1, this might be an exemplary moment of *purposeful beauty*. Clearly different touch moments might have different degrees of technique and expressiveness. A health professional might take a person's blood with a sense of calm, lightness of touch and effortless technique that meets the need for attention to the wellbeing of the patient and perhaps responds to a degree of anxiety on their part. This might be differentiated from the taking of blood with perfunctory attitude that functions technically but leaves a patient feeling cold and uncared for. Touch in care aesthetics, therefore, is an integrated set of practices, connected to other body practices of speech and movement, where at its best it is elegant and proficient, and where the boundary between technical with a degree of expressiveness and expressive with an element of technique is hard to distinguish. Again, touch is always a two-way experience, as expression and technique are also returned, so that, in Kosofsky Sedgwick's words, 'touch is always already to reach out [...] and always to understand other people or natural forces as having effectually done so before oneself' (2003: 14). At its best it can be part of a co-created moment, where it is sensed by all parties as an experience which has integrated elements of technique and expressivity.

The final point to make about touch is regarding the language used to discuss it. This is in some ways a small point to make, but in presenting a case for care aesthetics, it has additional significance. As a person touches another person, there is a tendency in analytical accounts to refer to this as a form of communication. Lennart Fredriksson, in his work on caring conversations in nurses, refers to caring touch as 'a form of non-verbal communication' (1999: 1171) and Classen argues 'touch has what could be called a vocabulary and a grammar' (2020: 13). In a world where the spoken and written word are the dominant modes of expression, this is hardly surprising. However, the argument here is that touch is reduced in its complexity if it is simply compared to communication, rather than expansively understanding it as an embodied inter-human practice. If we focus instead on touch as an important element of aesthetic experience, we have an alternative which is to see it as productive of relationships and a flow of feelings that have indeterminate meaning. It is rare that a touch on the arm can have a single verbal referent, such as 'Good morning', and therefore it does not speak in any predictable way. Classen, in fact, challenges her own assertion by suggesting that because of touch's immediacy 'language seems too formal and linear a model' (2020: 13), which is the exact point being made here. Tactile aesthetics, in Classen's terms, are part of care aesthetics, and exist as an integrated element of the experience that creates resonances and connections between people, which need a subtle language of appreciation and analysis. Touch cannot be explained as a mere substitute for talk.

Emotional and affective labour

If touch can be part of a care aesthetic experience and exists as a sub-category of practice within what is called bodywork, it can also be part of the broader analytical categories of emotional or affective labour. The original definition of emotional labour, developed by feminist sociologist Arlie Hochschild, explained it as 'the induction or suppression of feeling' to produce a sense in another person of being looked after (1983: 7). It is, thus, a concept connected to care and bodywork but also with a different focus. Hochschild's original account came from her study of flight attendants and how they managed their emotional repertoire in a job where their emotions were integral to the execution of their daily tasks. While Hochschild's theories have been applied to care by her (2003) and in the context of nursing by Pam Smith (2012), these uses raise questions for the case for care aesthetics. The first point to make is a brief one and repeats the argument above about bodywork. It is simply that the expression *emotional labour*, while helpful for focusing on the demands placed on many contemporary forms of employment, when applied to care, once again directs attention to one person in the caring relationship and does not sufficiently examine how care is reciprocal. If labour is the category of analysis, what is the response of the patient, client, elderly resident, and so forth? Of course, the airline passenger responds, but the case here is that a health and social care interaction is not captured sufficiently by a focus on the labour of one person. This is also the case with the related concept of *affective* labour discussed below. As expressed by Julia Twigg, emotional work is in fact 'never just one-way, and caring creates ties and bonds of affection that act back on the workers' (2002: 164). In the language of this chapter, ties and bonds of affection that touch back to the worker, are part of care aesthetics and need a rounded mode of analysis that does not leave one party out.

The second issue relates to the assumptions about 'labour' and what Hochschild calls the 'management of appearance', which while presented as descriptive of certain practices, can contain an implicit negative. Twigg in her work on bathing expresses an appreciation for the concept of emotional labour because it avoids the 'halo effect' of care (2002: 161) but the counter here is that in effect it produces the opposite, that is a negative 'halo'. Hochschild was explaining emotional labour as a process of managing feelings to 'sustain an outward appearance' (1983: 7) which is recognisable to many care workers as they complete the exhausting demands of shifts in hospitals or community settings. This is an important critique to appreciate the demands placed on many people working in the care sector. However, this does not capture the full sensory complexity of the work. Smith herself doubts emotional labour is a complete account, and, in fact, notes how it might belittle the notion of vocation that does still exist in many caring professionals' lexicon. While there are dangers in naturalising the desire to care, particularly as a propensity of women where the demand to care is so heavily weighted, there needs to be a way to recognise and not simply deny the sense of a 'call' to care that is reported by staff working in these contexts. This can be illustrated particularly through the choice of the word *appearance* which suggests an element of performance, or an artificially created front, masking the hidden emotional state of the worker. While many professions acknowledge a maintenance of a certain way of being at work as part of labour practices, in the health professions it is less satisfactory to create this division of *really* caring from *merely appearing* to care. There is managing care, so a person might sustain their engagement in the demands of their role, and this might be a struggle or done with ease but *appearing to care* does not capture the full experience of embodied care work.

While Twigg endorses emotional labour in her analysis, she later questions its applicability when showing how carers themselves discuss their work. In reporting on a study of a social services workforce, she explains how it became clear that 'home helps had higher levels of satisfaction in relation to nearly all aspects of their work than social workers, managers or residential staff' (2002: 126). Their involvement in home based intimate care, that is bodywork and emotional labour understood here, in fact led to higher degrees of satisfaction compared to those that were more distant from their patients or clients. Similarly, in a quotation that for me perfectly captures my caution with the concept of emotional labour, she reports the recurring problems in 'the analysis of service work that aspects that academics identify as exploitative are often enjoyed and valued by the workers; and one of the attractions of service work for many people is precisely the human interaction' (Ibid: 162). Emotional labour, a concept whose starting point is the identification of a problematic relation and the struggle to maintain the mask of appearing to care, meets care staff who value their work in a way that is not captured within the negative connotations of the term. Twigg in her more recent work on the body in health and social work, acknowledges this complexity by showing how 'not all the emotional aspects of body work are negative' and in fact 'emotion can also make body work worthwhile, meaningful and rewarding' (2011: 462). This perspective acknowledges that care work is demanding, and too often poorly paid and undervalued, but insists also that there is a reward in the quality of the relational experiences to which staff draw attention. By applying the framework of emotional labour to care, we create a vision of a nurse struggling with the demand to sustain an outwards appearance for the sake of their employment, when in fact carers report that it is the emotional engagement which is a valued part of their practice. It might be that other demands, the less embodied technical or managerial tasks, that are the focus of disquiet. This position accepts the labour as difficult but rejects the simplicity of the mask metaphor. It might be that the emotional labour is the *real*, and technical competence the 'mask' that a health professional struggles to manage. Technical labour might be the problem, with sensory and embodied practices being where satisfaction can be found.

The ambivalence expressed here, where the emotional or affective elements of a working practice, can be both hard to manage yet also a source of pleasure and reward, is noted in the work of Michael Hardt (1999) and with Antonio Negri in their analysis of 'affective labor' (2004). There is of course an overlap between Hardt's description of the rise in 'immaterial' labour that 'produces an immaterial good, such as a service, knowledge or communication' (1999: 94) and the work of Hochschild. The difference, however, is that he sees a possibility in a form of 'biopower from below' (Ibid: 100) where affective labour produces 'social networks, forms of community' and even the 'feeling of ease, well-being, satisfaction, excitement, passion' (Ibid: 96). The case for care aesthetics is that the creation of sensorily rich experiences of care, a form of affective labour in Hardt's terms, can exceed the expectations for care made in certain settings. Helen Nicholson echoes this point by arguing that affective labour should not be seen automatically as negative, but for the 'creative opportunities it generates, both artistically and socially' (2017: 107). The very immateriality of care means that it often exceeds the boundaries placed upon it. As the examples at the top of the chapter demonstrated, staff members at times commit to dynamic caring practices beyond the specific demands of their jobs or that can appear 'surprising' in the contexts of their work. While affective labour still places emphasis on the work undertaken by the carer, the point to emphasise is that it is an important concept for demonstrating the scope of a practice that is at times a form of affective work from below, surprising, resisting or creating caring encounters *despite* the demands of a context. It is hard to regulate the emotion, and thus the affect of caring labour, and this in turn creates a potential for it to exceed its limits and disrupt the negative assumptions academics have brought in their analysis of it.

The care encounter

A care aesthetics approach draws on the concepts of bodywork, and emotional and affective labour, but focuses on the care moment to value how carers and the cared for experience the emotions, sensations and relations that emerge across it.

It allows embodied care to be potentially rewarding experience for all parties, often in spite of the difficulties of the contexts in which it is undertaken. One mode of analysis that provides a framework for analysing care practices, that avoids some of the problems of one-sidedness outlined above, is considering the interaction as a 'caring encounter' (Cooper, 2001: 80). This connects to the idea of aesthetic *experience* outlined in Chapter 1, where the focus becomes a moment as it progresses across time, and includes all those present, their relations to each other and to the physical environment (from the smallest objects, to the built structures of a health care facility). Scholars in nursing and dementia studies take this approach through the idea of the 'experience in the moment' (Chinn and Watson, 1994: 24), which is presented as the appropriate unit of analysis because through close examination it can reveal the complexities of the interactions that take place across a relatively small amount of time. This mode of analysis draws attention to short exchanges to illustrate the importance of intimate qualities of what John Keady and colleagues call 'being in the moment' with 'the person living with dementia positioned as an active, creative contributor' (2020: 5). The effect of this focus and 'attentiveness to the extraordinary moments of an encounter' (Ibid: 2), is that a researcher or practitioner can become aware of the nuances of the 'relational, embodied and multi-sensory' (Ibid: 7) elements that are distributed across the experience, without an automatic sense of them being rewarding or exploitative. The language here suggests that being in the moment, being open to appreciation of the extraordinary in the everyday in the language of everyday aesthetics touched upon in Chapter 1, and to be examined further in the following chapter, requires a certain craft. Of course, in light of the concern expressed above with the notion of the art or craft of care, while a staff member might bring the attentiveness and skill, the experience is only realised in its richness and complexity through the contributions of all those present. According to the definition from Keady and colleagues in their study of *moments* across multiple dementia studies projects, it had a 'personal significance, meaning and worth' for those involved and importantly 'is both situational and autobiographical and can exist in a fleeting moment or for longer periods of time' (Ibid). In the focus on the smallest moment of interaction, we discover 'the fine-grained texture in everyday human-to-human relationships' (Ibid: 3), for example, when a patient responds in an unfamiliar way or demonstrates behaviour that offers a glimpse of memories or capacities that have not been revealed before. These moments, textured, multi-sensory and relational have, therefore, an aesthetics. They are not only an ideal unit of analysis to acknowledge the lived experience of people with dementia with a precision and respect to patients' capacities but also appropriate for close analysis of care aesthetics in action.

The fleeting nature of care encounters should not diminish their significance. As the different examples in Keady and colleagues' discussion of moments in dementia care demonstrate, they in fact offer a cumulative picture where 'moments can be positioned and linked together to provide a more holistic understanding of lived experience' (Ibid: 18). The section that follows will offer

a brief account of two care practices, hair styling and bathing, that in their execution produce moments that are significant in the lives of people in caring
relations. Following the emphasis of Keady and colleagues above, each is linked
to the care of the elderly. The intention of this focus is to follow the ethos of
Pam Smith's work on the labour of nursing that is 'about making the little things
big' (2012: xv). Directing the analysis to that which is deemed less significant or
worthy of attention is precisely the ambition of care aesthetics, as it seeks to value
those elements of the caring encounter that are too often ignored. What Smith
calls the 'little things' or 'gestures of caring' in fact 'slip unnoticed in the daily
routines and hustle and bustle of institutional life' (Ibid: 2) and the aim here is to
notice how they are crucial to the success of care in these contexts. Attention to
the care of the elderly is particularly important because, as discussed above, the
focus on the smallest moment might reveal aspects of their capacity and worth
that is too often overlooked. In an appropriate critique of the traditional focus
in hospital settings, Smith sums this up by arguing that 'on the elderly ward, the
high-tech heroics were set aside and the little things became all important' (Ibid:
1). The emphasis of care aesthetics is unashamedly championing the heroics of
the everyday gestures of care – 'little things such as dressing in their own clothes,
manicuring their nails, making sure their hearing aids worked and their glasses
were clean' (Ibid) – encounters of extraordinary importance, and sensory significance in the lives of those involved.

Hair care

Hair styling in care settings is a useful site for a care aesthetic analysis and the
comments here connect to the concerns raised about dressing in care settings
raised in Chapter 2. It is a practical activity, it is built around an encounter
between stylist and client, it involves bodywork, and it includes a complex set
of sensory demands and visual expectations. Twigg and Martin explain that 'the
close and ongoing relations between hairdressers and their clients might be uti-
lized as the new frontline of healthcare' (2015: 144) and I would add that it is
also a frontline between care and aesthetics. A stylist who visits a care home or
the home of an elderly person is undertaking a practice in which aesthetics and
care are interwoven. Similarly, like the process of dressing an elderly patient or
client, it is one where there can be tensions between visual expectations and
care needs. This relationship has been expertly documented in the project 'Hair
and Care' led by nursing scholars Sarah Campbell and Richard Ward which
developed an ethnographic study of a salon in a care home and the practices and
care encounters that took place there. This project appears in one of the quotations at the beginning of this chapter. While they do not use the expression
'care aesthetics', this project is an exemplary case of research that takes seriously
the aesthetics of the experiences they documented. In a series of publications
(Ward, Campbell, and Keady, 2014; Ward, Campbell and Keady, 2016a; Ward,
Campbell and Keady, 2016b), the authors illustrate how hair care in this setting

can be minutely attuned to the demands of the environment, the desires of the clients, and the skills of the stylists. In the words of the earlier quotation, this is a 'thermal, haptic and multi-sensory experience' involving both 'touch and talk' (2016a: 1293). This was not 'high-tech heroics', in Smith's language, but still involved highly skilled interactions including intimate body work, awareness of space, verbal communication and attention to the dignity of the elderly clients. While discussing hair styling in terms of aesthetics we might imagine that 'it was the suitably coiffed and neatly dressed "end product" of this work that was subject to scrutiny within the care system' (Ward et al, 2016a: 1288), in fact across the writing on this project, the researchers document an interplay of the final appearance and the process by which it is achieved. 'Hair and Care' acknowledged the significance of the end point in hair styling but gave even greater attention to the 'process of "doing appearance"' which for them was understood as a 'culturally and subjectively meaningful set of on-going practices that are integral to our identity and biographical selves' (Ward et al, 2016b: 399). There is, thus, an aesthetics of the hair care process and experience which is documented in their project, summed up in the expression 'sink work' (Ward et al, 2016a: 1293). They show how that process was involved in shaping identity, including as it did 'notions of pampering and sensual pleasure that are reinforced through one-to-one engagement' (Ward et al, 2016b: 404). Hair styling in this care home salon, therefore, was a practice that combined sensory pleasure and attentive care, making it an important example of what a *positive* care aesthetic experience might be.

In Campbell and Ward's work, they also documented a resistant quality of the salon experience as the stylists sought to counter some of the negative stereotypes of beauty and the ageing body in their work. The appointments in the salon involved a challenge to expectations of both the client and often the wider care home as a demonstration of the importance of this type of 'pampering'. When one of the hairdressers in the project 'hailed each newly arrived client with a promise of transformation' with the announcement '[g]onna make yer gorgeous!' (2016b: 401), we see a delight in the outcome of the endeavour, but crucially a sense that it is the process of 'making' that will shape the significance of the moment. There is a balance here between what Ward and colleagues refer to 'looking good' and 'feeling good' (Ibid: 406) that echoes the concerns raised in Chapter 2 about whether social care-based discussions of 'aesthetics of care' are in fact only discussing the visual. In Ward and colleagues work this was not the case, and in fact the relationships in the salon had to be understood as part of a process through which the 'good look' was created over time, and the whole experience, up to the 'gorgeous' result, engendered a sense of wellbeing and pride. Hairstyling, as pampering, and hair style as the 'good looking' outcome, are imbricated in an aesthetic caring process that is not reduced to the final reveal in the mirror. It is the greeting as a client arrives, the conversation during the process, the gentle washing of hair, the cutting, brushing, colouring and setting towards the end, and then the parting and complementing that create a total care aesthetic, time-based process. This is a 'moment' that has shifting sensory, auditory, and visual elements that tack in and out across the experience, shaping it as simultaneously a 'feeling good' and 'looking good' encounter.

Bathing

Like hair, the process of bathing is one that involves both a sensory experience and attention to expectations of the final outcome. The delicacy of this process is, of course, heightened when a person requires support to undertake what has been in the past a deeply personal and private process. Bathing is somewhat different from hair styling, and the dressing discussed in Chapter 2, because it has no automatic and explicit 'visual' aesthetic register. It is, of course, about cleanliness (which as Twigg shows so adeptly, is a historically changing concept) but it is also a sensory experience with task-based elements, making it relevant for the type of aesthetics being outlined here. In one of the book's opening vignettes, there was a description of a bathing moment as an example of one of the types of encounter care aesthetics was seeking to discuss. Julia Twigg's pioneering book, *Bathing: the body and community care* (2002), demonstrates both the importance of understanding many of the potential subtle pleasures in this sensory experience, and yet also how it can be difficult or troubling. The crux here is that a focus upon bathing as an aesthetic experience helps illustrate the delicacies of multi-sensory negotiation that need to take place in intimate body-work, and of course this has echoes in the analysis of the intimate *foot washing* by Adrian Howells in Chapter 3. Rovithis Michalis, in her review of the concept of *nursing as art*, saw bathing as exemplifying that artistry because it 'involves more than simplified mechanical practicable work' (2002: 4). Compared to relatives and other informal carers, in her view, nurses have a particular 'emotional art of caring' that can 'establish the trust between her and the patient' (Ibid). This is not guaranteed, however, and in fact the aesthetics of the bathing moment is less predictable and liable to be both pleasurable or uncomfortable, depending on the interrelation between the person doing bathing, the person being bathed, the context in which it occurs, and the time taken in the process. Thinking through this as an aesthetic encounter allows us to point to the complexities of the interrelations, the touch, the spoken word, the use of space, and how these intersect to produce the affective shape of the event. Twigg demonstrates how for some clients in her account of the bodywork of homecare workers, bathing in fact got in the way of a successful relationship with their carer, as the physical intimacies changed the dynamic of an interaction that was based more typically on conversation and company (2002: 70). It was the awareness of the home space, and the demands and desires of the client, and responding to these with sensitivity that determined whether the bathing was tolerated or enjoyed. It is perhaps noticeable in the debates about whether a care worker should use plastic gloves in bathing a client (and the majority do), that this was less about notions of hygiene and more about a dialogue with a client and a management of the expectations of professionalism. Bathing had a 'tactile aesthetics' that had to be negotiated with the expectations of both client and carer.

While there is an aesthetics of the bathing that cannot be automatically designated 'positive' or 'negative', in Twigg's account there are times where the pleasure of bathing as a co-created moment between the two people is emphasised. Clearly needing a carer to support bathing can produce a sense of loss from what for many was a private moment of calm or relaxation. However, there were examples where some of those sensations could be retrieved. Twigg explains that 'while bathing could never be quite what it had been, there was still some sensuous enjoyment to be had from it, and in the company of careworkers whom they liked, was a source of pleasure and human contact' (Ibid: 75). This indicates that it was the human relation prior to the bathing that needed to be in place to allow the moment to have this quality. Here bodywork that is connected to care, crosses into those that focus on 'body-pleasing and body-enhancing trades' (Ibid: 158), once again indicating how it is difficult to disentangle technical, therapeutic or expressive touch practices. A bathing care relationship, therefore, could still involve 'aspects of pleasure and sensuousness–the feeling of water being poured over the person, the luxury of shower foam, the warmth and lightness of the water' (Ibid). In the language of care aesthetics, it was an experience that required attentiveness and craft on behalf of the carer, an environment that allowed for the encounter to be realised successfully, and a recipient of the care to be an active, mutually recognised contributor. One of Twigg's care worker informants explained how creating this intimate space was not a given, but was a difficult process, that in particular involved a certain ability to create 'a time apart' (Ibid: 103). For her, bathing required the 'creation of a bounded space in which time stands still' where you could be in peace with somebody 'sharing that intimacy and cutting through the chaos of every day' (Ibid: 104). In a beautifully expressed summary of this moment, one of the elderly clients referred to this moment as the 'rose of my week' (Ibid: 103) again illustrating the potential for a delicate and pleasurable encounter to be realised in this moment. While it is important to emphasise that we should not overlook the difficulties of the intimate bathing moment in a care relationship, and these are real for both the overstretched worker and vulnerable client, we need to capture those elements of the relationship that can permit it to be articulated as a *rose*. It can have a quality, and perhaps by drawing attention to this care aesthetic, we might explore how having such a quality could be more predictable, that is a more common experience for both carer and cared for. Of course, there is the important analysis that points to bathing having potential for being represented by far less optimistic metaphors, but care aesthetics, when emphasising the positive, is a concerted search for that *rose*.

Place and time

Two elements that contribute to the possibility of bathing being experienced as dignifying and pleasurable, are related to the relationship between time taken and the place of its execution. Twigg referred to bathing as a 'time apart' and her care worker informant called the process of starting to bathe an elderly client as 'like entering an inarticulate space' (Ibid: 104). The final two sections of this chapter explore these elements by moving away from micro encounters to examine the importance of space, the environment in which a care encounter takes place, and how care is experienced temporally. While the aesthetics of care is understood within and between all those elements that make up a care experience, up to this point, there has been a greater focus on the inter-human relations that are particularly vital to it. These are of course imbricated within certain physical components, from the shape of the smallest needles, comfort of beds and linen, to the structure of wards, heating and light systems, and architecture of health and social care settings. Similarly, these experiences emerge within time-based patterns of shifts, hourly pay, cultural and managerial notions of efficiency and timeliness, and then broader rhythms of nights, days, weeks, and the changing seasons. These are not presented as external determining factors but seen as working in and through people, extending and contracting the possibilities of body practices and one's affective labour, and being realised in how they move, relate, and inhabit the places and times of their actions.

One way of describing the environment of health care in an aesthetic register comes from design, and the assertion that 'compassionate design of environments' can help 'the mutual recovery of all communities' (Crawford et al, 2015: 148). While this might be, according to Moss, a 'neglected or undervalued field' (2020: 431), there is a well-documented view that care needs to be considered not only as an interhuman practice but also in 'the context of green spaces and beautiful but ergonomic design' (Hanlon et al, 2012: 3196). Moss' critique of the 'aesthetics of deprivation', for example, is primarily directed towards greater attention to the décor, colour, and physical presentation of health care settings (2020: 434). One limit in these accounts, however, is that these attributes are viewed as giving 'a clue as to whether [they] meet the well-being of residents' or 'give an impression of insensitivity or indifference to the patients' (Ibid). The perspective here is that environmental aspects of a care setting are not signals of the quality of care, much like the dressing of a resident cannot be taken as a straightforward, visual surrogate for the quality of care. The environment needs to be understood as actively creating the care that is possible in any particular settings, and both affecting and being affected by the relationships that take place within it. This is well expressed in the nuanced account of the salon in Ward and colleagues Hair and Care project, where physical elements of the room would be rearranged by the stylists so that they then 'took on properties' that then stimulated new meanings and orientations for those present (2016a: 1292). For them rather than a static environment 'giving an impression' of the quality of care, 'certain objects and material features played a distinctive part in the theatre of body work that extended well beyond their functional purpose' (Ibid). This is suggestive of a more fluid, interactive process between people and environment. For a full account of care aesthetics, therefore, the site must be understood to take an active role in the unfolding of a sensory experience. The analysis therefore borrows from the writing of care geographers who refer less to an environment and instead to the idea of a caringscape that is made up of 'interactive, processual experiences' that make care possible (Bowlby et al, 2010: 247).

Ward and colleagues refer to their salon as a 'micro-site' (Ibid) and Twigg and Martin refer to care contexts as the 'materialized microcosmic world' (2015: 170), particularly when talking about the delicate exchanges between the many physical and human elements that shape an experience of bathing. What is important for an understanding of the environment in care aesthetics, however, is that where the human ends and the material world begins is difficult to discern. So, by way of example, gloves, needles, walking sticks, grab bars, and scalpels, extend from and in turn fold back into capacities of the body. By extension, the micro cannot be disaggregated from macro environmental demands with any precision. Twigg and Martin point out that 'intimate assemblage of spaces and relationships [...] intersect with macro-worlds of health, safety, social support and quality of life' (Ibid). When discussing the design of dementia environments, Twigg and Martin call this a 'complicity between place and the embodiment of history' (Ibid: 177), and it is this fluid relationship between practices of a different scale that is important to recognise. In effect we can sense the macro in micro behaviours, and the weight of a built environment can shape the smallest of intimate interactions. The 'assemblage' of an aesthetic experience is an imbrication of space and relationships, with care practices flowing across and between different scales of affective, always sensory environmental configurations. The gentle push of a person in a wheelchair down a hospital corridor, meets lumps in the floor, brilliant whites on walls, buzzing electric lights, the friendly greetings of cleaners, the brusque walk by of stressed staff, the coffee machine that cannot be fed coins by a person in a wheelchair, and then a warm embrace of the family member. Where physical environment begins and ends, where health policy acts on the situation or is changed by it, and where people experience care because of or in spite of the multiple elements of its spatial arrangements, are difficult to disentangle. Care aesthetics seeks to track that experience, that journey down a corridor, for the multiple, intersecting sensory elements and show how at times they enhance a lived experience, and of course how they also diminish it.

One of the most famous examples of this micro attention to the relationship between people and space in the context of health care is in the Maggie's Centre movement in the UK. These are purpose-built centres and integrated gardens, more often than not in the grounds of hospitals, for the care of people undertaking cancer treatment and their families. Inspired by the experience of Maggie Keswick Jencks, and her treatment for breast cancer, the organisation has now pioneered the development and design of numerous centres that offer support for people in treatment, with a place of respite, relaxation, and where needed advice or company. The first was opened in Edinburgh in 1996, and at time of writing in 2022 there are twenty-four in the UK and three more internationally. While these beautiful spaces deserve much more detailed study from the perspective of care aesthetics, they illustrate the argument here because the buildings are not framed as passive indicators of the quality of care, but as productive partners in its realisation. In the Maggie's 'Architecture and Landscape Brief' there is a clear sense that the buildings have agency, and they aim 'to coax people out of their feeling of isolation and to help them feel less locked in' (MALB, 2020: 5). These are spaces that should be addressing cancer patients, 'saluting the magnitude of the challenge they are facing' and 'they should be beautiful' (Ibid: 4). It is hard to imagine a care home that would use the language of saluting its residents, or a ward being designed to salute its patients. In Maggie's Centres, however, there is a vision of an environment that acts with people and is part of the process of recovery as an engaged partner. The practice proposed by the design brief and evidenced in the different buildings that now exists across the UK is of a health care setting not as a container but as a collaborator, co-creating a lived experience through the space and the interpersonal encounters made possible by it. In Bowlby and colleagues' discussion of the Maggie's Centres, they articulate this as a 'relationships between the physical form of such spaces, their environmental characteristics, and the social activities that constitute them' (2010: 2646). They absolutely stand against an aesthetics of deprivation, but not merely as a visual signal demonstrating the quality of care of a particular hospital, but rather as an integral part of its creation.

It is notable in the briefing for architects of new Maggie's Centres, that it is not only the environment that is active in the care for the people that move through and find a place within them but also a sense of a new arrangement of time. This is through a spatial configuration that encourages those within it to find their own pace and reorientate themselves from the temporal demands of the hospital experience of endless appointments and diarised procedures. Time is important for the Maggie's centres' understanding of care, and in many ways, it has been one of the unspoken elements across many of the practices discussed here. The chapter opened with an account of the care of my colleague Antoine, and how his physiotherapist was able to treat him with such artfulness because her practice existed beyond the usual demands of the economies of time in a private hospital. The chapter concludes by returning to time, to notions of the quick and the slow, the calm and the rushed, the pressurised and the relaxed, to note that it has an embodied, sensory aspect that is vital to an understanding of care aesthetics. This can be seen in Moss' category of 'aesthetics deprivation' where she refers to clinics that are designed both carelessly and 'in haste' (2020: 434). However, the significance of that 'in haste' is greater than an account of rushed design, because it is indicative of a more fundamental conflict between different understandings of the organisation of care work. Bunting has demonstrated how one of the central binds in contemporary care is that 'carers find themselves caught between clock-based time and task-based time' (2020: 47), where the clock divides time into predictable and quantifiable portions, but tasks, especially in embodied care, have a rhythm that cannot be paced out in precise minutes. The effect is that adequate care often cannot be executed to the quality a carer might hope due to the demands of a contract based on strict allocations of increasingly limited time periods. Bunting explains the word 'nursing' etymologically, as in 'nursing a glass of brandy' and how it 'speaks of attentiveness and a slow pace' (Ibid: 102). This is a pace which is increasingly under pressure in many health and social care contexts. Hochschild actually sets care against the demand for 'speed-up' suggesting that the organisation of care by the clock means that it is no longer the work of a 'caring nurse' (2012: xiv). While this opposition is perhaps too strong, it is clear that many of the component parts of caring do not fit easily into a strictly clock-based framework. When Hochschild is discussing 'the commercialization of intimate life' (the title of her 2003 book), it is the way that the commercial organises and comes to dominate time that is the problem for care. Her concern is that bodywork will always struggle to be contained within precisely codified timed boundaries. Care time, such as bathing, changing dressings, and of course building relationships, is always unpredictable and subject to the particularities of the people involved and the context in which it happens. A 'regulatory regime' in the words of Twigg, where people are 'fed, bathed, toileted according to schedule' interrupts an alternative embodied rhythm that rarely fits a timetable in this way. While clock-based time does not make quality care impossible, the prevalence of strict time codes across multiple commercial relations of care does ensure that carers and the people they care for, are constantly negotiating care experiences between different time signatures. The greater the prescriptions of clock-based time, the more the rhythm of an interhuman care process becomes constrained or disturbed.

This tension between sped up managed time and the prescribed routines of care 'according to schedule', has led to demands for a slowing down of care, both as a way of improving its execution, and resisting the *commercialisation of intimate life*. In setting this demand alongside the mission of the Maggie's centres for a completely new way of experiencing an environment during a period of illness, we can start to see how a more responsive, fluid and interactive relation between care and the time it takes and the spaces in which it is realised, is in fact a much broader proposal for a systematic reimagination of care. This brings this chapter full circle to thinking how artful care might be realised not only in the micro-relations between caring professionals and their clients and patients, but in the sense of seeing them as part of a larger ecosystem or culture of care, that lives in and through their work but also shapes much broader systems of support across a range of contemporary contexts. And into this mix, as I mentioned at the top of this chapter, we need to reintroduce the artists and consider what roles they might take in bringing their practices of careful art alongside the artful care that exists in many care settings. Theatre scholar Nicola Hatton has proposed that the key to successful practice of artists in care homes is slowing down and attending 'creatively to the different temporalities of everyday life in a care home' (2020: 96). Her work is significant both for the modesty of her proposition that fits with the argument here that artists need to appreciate the existing aesthetics of the care context in which they work, but, also, she is proposing an attentiveness to the particular temporal particularities of people living with dementia. Hers is a call for an in tune and slowed down practice. The aesthetic metaphor of 'in tune' here is, of course, deliberate. Nurses, homecare workers, health professionals and artists working in health settings, create an aesthetically rich experience that is attuned to needs, responsive to an environment, but at times resistant to the rhythms and constraints that diminish the life experiences of those living in those settings.

Chapter 4 has explored care aesthetics in health and social care settings. How it might take the craft, or art, of a care worker in tandem with the response of the person being cared for and the contingencies of the context they inhabit, to create aesthetically rich, sensorily dynamic caring experiences. It has shifted attention from the art of nursing, to a more embedded version of the care experience that is a fluid interchange of environment, time, and the responsiveness of all parties to the moment. It has illustrated how aesthetic deprivation in care contexts and the increasing demands on carers time has created diminished experiences of care and yet care workers have also continued, in partnership with those that they care for, to create aesthetically 'positive' encounters. This is evidenced in micro worlds of bodywork, which while being definitively emotionally laborious can also involve carers finding pleasure in building relationships with patients and clients. Drawing this chapter to an end, we start to see how trying to find positive care aesthetic experiences will involve artists and creative people in partnership with the care environments, in a way that Basting envisaged when she called for the pouring of creativity 'into the water of an organization so it spread through its systems to all its staff, the elders, and their families' (2020: 234). This might be a description of Maggie's Centres which in effect pour a new way of operating into the heart of a hospital complex and perhaps start a process of changing practices across it. Extending this metaphor, the next question to ask might be what happens when that spread cannot be contained in an organisation, and the commitment transfers into the water ways, leaking into different aspects of our everyday lives. The next chapter takes this forward, and moves out of the immediate formal care setting, to ask how might care aesthetics meet some of the demands of the everyday. How does a more general aesthetic of deprivation, that is experienced in multiply ways by different communities, become addressed if we seek to develop new forms of everyday care aesthetics?

5

Everyday care aesthetics

When I first started writing on *care aesthetics*, one aim was to question the boundaries in applied theatre or socially engaged arts between, on the one hand, the artists who had the capacity for operating in an aesthetic register and, on the other, the social, education and health workers who operated in a register of care. I became interested in how artists demonstrated care in their work whether through attention to actors and participants, focus on objects, involvement of communities, or design of spaces. Questioning arts practices through the prism of care revealed new dynamics and tensions in some of the claims that were made. Similarly, I was interested in when social, health, or care workers demonstrated an artistry or craft in their work: when they practiced with a certain attention to aesthetics. I wanted to know what it might mean to critique care practices for their lack of attention to a sensory experience or when they were executed without an aesthetic sensibility.

In seeking to query this boundary *care aesthetics* was trying to imagine practices which were both caring and aesthetic without assuming who was automatically entitled to the designation 'carer' or 'artist'. So, the physiotherapist could demonstrate *care aesthetics* in her work with a patient, as her touch and hold exhibited a certain craft, and the experience between patient and therapist involved a certain heightened sensory quality. Similarly, a neighbour may cook a meal for an isolated friend which demonstrated her love and affection for them. A social movement might be structured with a certain *care aesthetics* in the dynamic way it maintained bonds and support between its activists. A community association might shape a day centre for its elderly members with attention to the look and feel of an environment that validated residents' sense of worth and was in turn appreciated for how it operated with a supportive sense of place. Care aesthetics was trying to get away from the idea that the socially engaged arts were about places empty of aesthetics inviting the artists into their midst to invigorate them

DOI: 10.4324/9781003260066-8

with joy, play and craft, with a model, instead, that suggested there is care aesthetics in many different parts of our lives. We need to sustain our ability to care for each other, for our communities and for the worlds in which we live with great craft and skill without thinking that only those with the formal title 'artist' can provide this. Of course, artists can and do provide rich *care aesthetic* experiences, but we need to democratise who is valued for their aesthetic work and recognise the skills of multiple practitioners and professionals. We also need to be reminded that an experience is made by all those involved in a moment, and not only those with 'care' or 'artistic' responsibilities. When the times in which we live value the technical and managerial over the embodied and affective, *care aesthetics* is a demand for a slower, more human-centred relational focus for acts of care. As mentioned at the end of the previous chapter, this is a perspective indebted to the work of Nicola Hatton in her demand for 'slower collaborations' and greater attunement to the patterns of daily life in artistic practice in elderly care home settings (2019: 96). Similarly, the argument is making a demand that in a world of extremes of lack of care, and the *ugliness* of poverty and discrimination, we need to improve the way we live together to ensure the damaging and unequal relations that dominate our worlds have a chance to be transformed. *Care aesthetics* is about the shape and feel of how we look *after* each other and how we look *out* for each other: it is about the art and craft of acting in solidarity.

In the last two chapters, these debates have been laid out in relation to arts, health, and social care contexts, but the final pages of the previous chapter hinted that the proposal of care aesthetics inevitably starts to shift beyond these contexts to bring a range of everyday practices under scrutiny. The deficits of care, particularly revealed during the Coronavirus pandemic, are not only experienced within the formal care sector, but are experienced across multiple areas of our lives. If as proposed in books such as Bunting's '*Labour of Love*' (2020) and the London-based Care Collective's '*Care Manifesto*' (2020), care inequalities are now a preeminent injustice structuring people's ability to lead fulfilling lives, the final chapter asks what implications this might have for a proposal for care aesthetics. What does an account of care aesthetics in the everyday reveal about practices that might challenge the current inequalities in care provision and start to shape a more careful and care-filled world?

The concluding chapter takes this question to make the case for, in Basting's words, *pouring creativity into the water* (2020: 234) so sensorially rich care aesthetic experiences become notable in multiple relations of mutual and community support. It will outline a definition of the everyday as an important site of social and political practice and return to the definitions of everyday aesthetics outlined in Chapter 1. It will then seek to transfer these approaches to a proposal for everyday care and highlight this orientation through the brief example of food and cooking, and then in everyday responses to the Coronavirus pandemic. The argument here is that in an event that has revealed terrible inadequacies in our care systems, there are important responses that illustrate care aesthetics in action. Of course, in many ways this is a return to the account of singing from balconies and clapping for carers made at the very beginning of the book. Finally, by way of conclusion, I will draw on my personal experience during the UK's extended lockdown, to make a case for how care aesthetics has become an important framework for some of my own care/art practices. As the final chapter of the book, there is, therefore, a tentative proposal for how care aesthetics might *pour* into our everyday lives with some suggestions for where practice and research in this area might develop.

The everyday

The everyday is invoked here not to create a special place that is designated as distinct from the formal or professional aspects of how we live. It is, according to anthropologist Sarah Pink, 'where we live our lives' (Pink, 2012: 30) and is used therefore to suggest a fluid relation between micro activities of managing those aspects of our lives we undertake to keep going and the institutions, conventions and social structures that surround us. In claiming the importance of the everyday, and suggesting it is a significant context for understanding the ethics and aesthetics of care, it is not, however, an alternative to the practices explored in the previous two chapters. It is rather an account of the continuum between them. We do not exercise care in an everyday, routine setting and then cross a precisely defined border to practice in a formal, institutional one. We are always and already interweaving the formal and informal in our lives. This is a position borrowed from feminist geographers who insist on an 'empirical inadequacy' of any dichotomy and argue, for example, that the 'private space of the home is enmeshed in the relations of the public sphere of production and civil society' (Bowlby et al, 2010: 1717). The professional and personal are folded into each other (perhaps complementary, perhaps in tension) and everyday tasks (shopping, cooking, childcare, family visits, meeting friends) tack back and forth between activities of public or professional importance (work, study, volunteering, campaigning, training). The perspective here is this interrelation ensures that the everyday involves a set of processes that are acutely important for the quality of our lives, and for many people the preeminent context through which they might act to maintain, repair, or improve them.

In her foreword to Marion Young's unfinished final work *Responsibility for Justice* (2010), Martha Nussbaum argues that we have witnessed the gradual erosion of the 'idea of collective responsibility' so that an 'individualist understanding of social relations' now dominates (Ibid: 9). She praises Young's work for trying to bring together an acceptance of the powerful structural inequalities that shape communities, with a continued commitment to a responsibility for people to take action to address those injustices. Young's work avoids the dichotomy between a perspective that locates all problems with a determining social structure and one that blames individuals for poor life outcomes. It argues instead for a renewal of a 'social connection model of responsibility' that is a forward-looking sense that individuals have 'an obligation to join with others [...]

in order to transform the structural processes to make their outcomes less unjust' (Ibid: 96). Rather than a retrospective politics that focuses on the events in the past that led to current inequalities and injustice, one that exists in the register of blame for past action or inaction, it argues for the solidarity of relationships 'among many people who recognize and take up shared responsibility' in the present or immediate future (Ibid: 121). For the purpose here, this perspective signals a focus on an everyday where those responsibilities are undertaken and where everyday solidarities, even in the smallest actions, start to shape people's lives. Historian Paul Ginsborg, in his work on everyday politics, refers to this as a process that seeks to 'build horizontal solidarities rather than vertical loyalties' (2005: 133) and the case here is that *joining with others*, in activities of everyday micro solidarity, demands an account of how that joining is crafted and experienced. It suggests that a consideration of the care aesthetics of Young's everyday collective responsibility might ensure more enduring and richly felt horizontal relations that contribute to making life more liveable and just.

The argument in Chapter 5, therefore, borrows Young's 'social connection model' but is adapting it to speak of how the connections are made, and what the taking of responsibility might look like in practice. Returning to Pink, she has expertly demonstrated how 'everyday life and activism are often studied in isolation from each other' where the 'everyday has tended to be associated with the mundane, the routine and the hidden' and activism on the other hand 'has been linked to the public, explicit, explosive, and sometimes even glamorous elements of political life' (2012: 4). In making the argument for everyday care aesthetics, this division is rejected to assert that there is an activism of the everyday, and the registers of care and aesthetics are vital for understanding it. The purpose here is to suggest that it might be hidden, but it is the place in which many people do enact solidarities by taking responsibility for building and developing their social connections. Crucially, in focusing her research on the everyday, Pink notes that to understand this form of everyday activity we need to explore 'ordinary ways of being' (Ibid: 14) which are revealed through 'sensory socialities of activism' (Ibid: 10). If the task according to Young is to connect to overcome atomised individualism, my case here will be that care aesthetics might be one way of understanding or framing the 'sensory sociality' of constructing and sustaining those connections.

One of the most famous theorists of everyday life was French philosopher, Michel de Certeau, particularly laid out in his seminal *The Practice of Everyday Life* (1984). The politics of the everyday for de Certeau involved people taking a degree of control of their material contexts using 'popular procedures' (Ibid: xiv) and the creation of 'an esthetics [sic] of tricks [...] an ethics of *tenacity*' (Ibid: 26. Italics in the original). His was a vision of the oppressed worker or citizen using guile, evasion and underhand tactics, in order to resist the dominance of the strong. De Certeau wrote of the eking out of an *in spite of* zone where survival was made possible by trickster ruses that evaded the reach of the more powerful. While this clearly chimes with the sensory sociality discussed above and is important for its willingness to permit the 'miniscule' and 'quotidian' (Ibid: xiv) as part of the complexity of political action, the emphasis here is somewhat different. In focusing on the everyday as a site for sociality, a place of connection or solidarities at the quotidian level, it is less the tenacity exhibited by the cleverly resistant individual that is the focus. Instead, it is more the process by which relations between people are built and strengthened. Understanding care as an act of solidarity in the everyday means attention is drawn to collaborative acts. These are daily routines of family, neighbourly and community interaction that develop micro interrelationships and enhance the bonds of care they provide for overcoming difficulties. It is less individual guile, and more communal endeavour that provides a bulwark against isolation and a sense of powerlessness. Human geographer, Kye Askins, in her work on geographies of care, has demonstrated these types of relations in her analysis of refugee support projects. Her account of 'a quiet politics that is enacted in initiating interpersonal relationships' (2014: 353) is exactly the register suggested here. This is a context in which care aesthetics might define the contours and sensations of an intimate politics of the everyday: one that takes the building of relations between groups and individuals as a process through which new sensorily rich, life enhancing solidarities can be formed. Clearly it might be practiced with a certain *tenacity* or *aesthetic of tricks*, but it is one done through collaborations, interactions and daily acts of living with others.

Everyday aesthetics

The aim here is not to repeat the comments on everyday aesthetics made in Chapter 1. As noted there, the field, particularly in the work of Yuriko Saito, opens a space for aesthetics in the daily activities of human to human and human to object interaction, that make it a fertile ground for developing the notion of care aesthetics. To make the claim that care as a practice could be understood aesthetically, the field of everyday aesthetics was important in demonstrating how aesthetic theory extended well beyond an appreciation of what was designated 'the arts' in any particular culture. There are two points to re-emphasise here. First, I acknowledged that the debate as to whether everyday aesthetics was drawing attention to the especially aesthetic within an everyday that was largely mundane and routine, or that it explained how even the underwhelming routine activities of daily life have their aesthetic, was not one I sought to resolve. Daily chores, for example cleaning the house, preparing a meal, or doing the laundry, have an aesthetic in that they deal with sensory perception, choices of look, feel and smell, involving both aesthetic decisions and resulting in aesthetic forms of appreciation. The sensory practices and conventions of, for example, cleanliness in any particular culture or period of history were referred to in Chapter 1 as a type of sensorium or sensory schema. Where I differed from Saito was that she deemed all of daily life, whatever its intensity, to have an everyday aesthetic, whereas I preferred to place greater attention on experiences in the everyday that provided a form of heightened aesthetic. The mundane chore, therefore, does have its aesthetics but I am making the case for *greater* attention to enhancements in aesthetic sensation and experience, as part of a project that is seeking to make everyday life richer and more sensorially rewarding. Everyday care of course might have a diminished, perfunctory, or even unpleasant aesthetic, but the case for care aesthetics is not content simply to describe those practices. It is also part of a critical project that argues that poor care results in injustices and it is therefore seeking to determine care practices where a heightened attention to aesthetics, to more rewarding and powerfully crafted experiences, make them more enriching and life enhancing. Following the arguments in the first part of the chapter, to increase the potential for social connection, for new models of 'sensory socialities of activism', and what I called affective solidarity in earlier chapters, we need to strengthen the aesthetic qualities of the everyday, particularly everyday interhuman relations. So, yes everyday aesthetics provides a sensory contour to multiple aspects of our lives, but everyday care aesthetics is also a project that demands heightened, richer, more dynamically crafted interhuman relations of care as a small part of the process of building 'horizontal solidarities'.

The second point to return to is that there is a tendency in Saito's work to view an openness or awareness of aesthetics of the everyday as a personal virtue that in turn leads to people making 'moral-aesthetic' judgements (2008: 208). While I agree with her demand that 'the distinction between the aesthetic and the moral is blurred' (Ibid: 238), she sees 'care, consideration, and thoughtfulness' (2017: 150) as virtues that are inherent qualities of an individual, even when they are cultivated by aesthetic means. As explained in Chapter 1, this can mean a judgement of others, their standing as individuals, being based on the aesthetics of their comportment or even attire. My position is slightly different and develops the point in the previous chapter that raised a concern about the limitation of the sole focus on the 'art of the nurse'. Rather than an attention to individual virtue, I see ethics and aesthetics as dependent on interpersonal relations, arising within the moment of an interhuman experience which can only be judged by those involved in that experience. The sense of a personally held virtue and then the capacity to judge others, is replaced with a care aesthetics in everyday settings the quality or meaning of which emerges and is realised by those present in the encounter. This is important here because the proposal is not about cultivating virtuousness or a capacity to judge practices that are 'morally-aesthetically' wanting. Drawing on Young's aspiration for a forward-looking politics of connective responsibility, the approach here is to advocate a collective responsibility for creating more life enhancing, creatively caring relations between people, that might help counter many of the inequalities and injustices that exist in contemporary communities. Everyday aesthetics as a field helps outline daily life as area of experience where that responsibility is enacted but it is one in which carefulness and the facilitation of more equitable social participation emerge through the experience and are not necessarily virtues inherent in individuals prior to the engagement.

Everyday care

The everyday, for this chapter, is therefore not a separate zone of experience from the areas discussed in Chapters 3 and 4. This is not a restatement of a division between public worlds of professional care and the private or domestic spaces on familial caring responsibilities. It endorses health geographer Christine Milligan's position that it is wrong to view 'the worlds of formal and informal care as discrete entities' (2016: 133) and instead agrees we should be exploring how care is manifested across landscapes that stretch 'from the home and community-based settings to the care home and beyond' (Ibid: 144). The chapter is, therefore, an attempt to expand care aesthetics to argue that the way we relate to others, the way we shape relations within our communities, extends outwards from what might be caring and artistic work in more formal settings. Similarly, the converse is also true so that practices at home, amongst neighbours and in communities extend back into more professional or vocational settings. It argues that aesthetically caring practices materialise and fold forward and backwards between different parts of our everyday.

In early work on care ethics, Nel Noddings made a distinction between what she called 'natural caring' and 'ethical caring' (2013: 198). The former referred to care that was unchosen, for example mother to child, and the latter was concerned with those practices 'where a decision was made to care' (Ibid). This difference in some way mirrors the potential for the focus here on the everyday to be understood as care that is part of familial obligation or one's inherent role as opposed to those that are formal or part of our public duties. The purpose here is to challenge this division, to argue that the embodied and sensory practice of care cannot fit neatly into the natural/ethical, or informal/formal, or even private/public divisions. The research in the previous chapter where carers explained how the bodywork they undertook was deemed to be a satisfying part of their work, illustrates that unchosen and chosen forms of care (for example, for a child rather than for a patient) in fact borrow from each other in terms of the feelings, practices and sensations they elicit. As Milligan writes, 'the physical nature of caring might change' but 'the affective elements remain' (Ibid: 123). Care is not automatically 'natural' to one setting and 'ethical' to another. It is shaped across personal capacities, previous experiences, and culturally learnt processes that then materialise in different ways in multiply different situations. An account of 'everyday care' therefore is not an argument about the care that takes place once someone leaves their job in a hospital and returns home, moving from ethical to natural care, but an argument for seeing the continuities (and of course discontinuities) in all our capacities to experience care in different moments across our lives.

The attempt to trouble this distinction is not to deny that there are differences, degrees of compulsion and control, or duty and desire in caring relationships, but to argue that these shift in unexpected ways and frequently not along the simple lines suggested by the dichotomies listed above. The focus here is how we might draw on the best creative, aesthetically dynamic caring practices in multiple moments, to ensure people are connected, cared for, and allowed to thrive. This might mean learning from neighbourhood-based mutual aid, micro processes of community, or even street-based support, and interfamily practices of childcare, as well as the best in patient advocacy, nursing practice, or a worker's embodied care of elders. Everyday care aesthetics asks the question how might the best care skills that are brought to one area of one's life, become an inspiration for another. How might the creative care in a drama project, for example, also inspire changes in the way we interact with people we encounter in our immediate communities? How might the way we check in on a neighbour, listening and giving time to his or her stories and concerns, inform a certain attentiveness in our engagement with students in our classes?

Everyday care aesthetics

Everyday care aesthetics is, therefore, meant to cast a wide net to include practices that might be thought peripheral and not significant for consideration when arts or care practitioners think about their practices. David Gauntlett on his work on craft refers to *everyday creativity* (2011: 221) and the expansive version of care aesthetics here idea borrows from his commitment to accounting for the daily acts of crafting that people demonstrate in many parts of their lives. The ambition is to consider the caring experiences that might be fostered through those craft acts but also pay fuller attention to the range of caring behaviours that people commit to in the course of living and working in different communities that are less obviously art or craft based. As with the rest of this book, the argument is that the everyday acts of building, maintaining and improving relations between people can be part of a creative practice. Saito captures this in her description of the way we 'we interact with others through handling of objects, tone of voice, facial expressions, and bodily movements, all of which are *aesthetics* factors' (2017: 179. Italics in the original). The outcome of these 'aesthetic factors' for her is an increase in 'kindness and caring' (Ibid: 178) which in turn can create an 'affable, convivial ambience' (Ibid: 50). While this might sound a touch genteel, an appeal to codes of behaviour demanding consensus and acquiescence, the perspective here is that acts with an aesthetic of care can start a process of mutual support and repair, and then perhaps be extended into practices of 'sensory socialities of activism' that might provide sustenance to communities under pressure. Strengthening inter-human sensory care, is not a proscriptive process of gradual adoption of 'beautiful manners' (Ibid: 180) but a practical endeavour of changing everyday carelessness and countering assumptions of inevitable individualism with multiple acts of locally based creative solidarity.

One place that this practical endeavour may be realised in through the way different communities make, share, and come together through eating and preparing food. As noted in Chapter 3, food can be a place that, in public health researcher Phil Hanlon's terms, ethics, science and aesthetics meet. He makes the case that in everyday contexts, it is hard to disentangle the functional and technical aspects of food preparation from how it performs as an expression of care or love (2016: 23). Of course, cooking and eating should not be understood romantically as a guaranteed site of fellowship as inequalities in labour, access to ingredients and food poverty structure how it is experienced in many families and communities. What I want to touch on here, however, is how while much of what Saito calls 'food aesthetics' (2017: 56) has a mundane yet still aesthetically important quality, it is in moments of difficulty and crisis that the preparation, distribution and sharing of food can take on particular importance. While food banks, soup kitchens, and emergency food aid should not be taken as the answers to injustice, they do provide important bulwarks against the worst in food-related inequality. What is significant is that food in these contexts is often not distributed in a perfunctory way but is done so with an exceptional attention to its quality, presentation, and the form through which it is donated. Of course, this is not always the case, but there are multiple examples where it is. It might be as simple as an organisation close to my neighbourhood in Manchester, UK, the Barlow Moor Community Association, who during the Coronavirus pandemic in 2020 and 2021 changed the way they delivered their services to move to 'remote befriending, cake and conversation' (2021: no page). The food was important, but it was embedded in micro acts of reaching out and ensuring people were less isolated. Similarly, the Manchester based organisation *Cracking Good Food* cooked over 85000 meals for people during the pandemic, again with a commitment to 'good food for all' that was simultaneously part of a commitment to tackling food poverty and waste (Calouste Gulbenkian Foundation, 2021: no page). There were numerous similar acts of community cooking during the pandemic, where local kitchens and community bakers not only provided sustenance to people in need but also produced food with a level of care and attention, that sought to project the sense that supporting others well should be done not just by the act of cooking, but through the aesthetics of the care brought to it. Returning to the argument above connected to Saito's advocacy of everyday aesthetics as one that includes the routine or mundane, the point about everyday care aesthetics, demonstrated often in food responses to crisis, is that people create it with a heightened aesthetic concern. A commitment that indicates that caring solidarity is magnified through greater attention – *beyond what might be functionally necessary* – to the quality, taste and form the food takes. As someone who personally witnessed a kitchen table covered in hundreds of cakes, muffins, cupcakes, and loaves, decorated and arranged with astounding care, colour, and sense of fun, I was constantly reminded during the pandemic that food was one place that an aesthetics of everyday care was realised.

Of course, in charitable settings such as these, the relationship of care has a power imbalance where benevolence can too easily drift into paternalism. While acknowledging this risk, following the 'social connection model of responsibility' from Young, the argument here is that awareness of structural factors in inequality, should not then absolve us from taking action to mitigate immediate needs that arise from it. In many ways, the case for care aesthetics contributes to this debate through insisting that the way that care and direct support is delivered in urgent, or emergency situations should not diminish people's dignity through an uncaring and patronising method of distribution. *Paternalism* has an aesthetic too: an embodied shape and feel through which it is realised, with expected patterns of gratitude and contrition. If we draw proper attention to the sensations of reciprocity, mutual respect and felt relations of trust, some of the difficulties of the unequal relationships in the aid world might be avoided. While, of course, this is not guaranteed, and my experience in conflict zones suggests that the aesthetics of aid are too rarely appreciated (Thompson, 2014), what follows is an example where food aid, aesthetics and care did come together.

The UK Non-Governmental Organisation Refugee Support was founded in 2016 in response to the refugee crisis in Europe and now operates predominantly with recently arrived refugee communities in Greece. The founders, John Sloan and Paul Hutchings, explain that they set up the organisation due to the careless and undignified way they had witnessed aid being delivered in the camps around Calais, in northern France. Their stories of random sized clothing been thrown *at* refugees off the back of a lorry, without thought as to what individuals might want or feel met their needs, could be called a practice with a negative care aesthetics as outlined in previous chapters. In an interview in the Guardian in 2018, Paul Hutchings asks the question as to how they might 'give people food and clothing without taking away their dignity' (Nayeri, 2018: no page). His solution was to focus on the way aid was delivered and in particular their vision was realised in the design of a shop in the camp where they were working. The ambition was for the space to look and feel like a community store and be a pleasant place to visit. The shop, once completed, distributed food, clothes and other provisions and allowed camp residents to purchase items through an agreed system of exchange. It was 'a well-designed, peaceful marketplace stocked with donations, where a person of note wouldn't be ashamed to shop' (Ibid) and significantly, when creating the shop, Hutchings spent time 'thinking of the aesthetics, whether people will like it' (Ibid). In a simple, almost surprised aside, the interviewer Dina Nayeri writes 'he cares that they *like* it' (Ibid: italics in the original). A solution to the problem of the undignified way that aid is distributed, a practice that can undermine a person's sense worth, is met with a focus on the aesthetics of the care by which the aid relation in exercised. The terrible situation facing many refugee communities in Europe is not overcome in this, but an aesthetic of care creates a micro practice of offering and maintaining their dignity at a time when it has been challenged by difficult experiences, direct threat, and poor treatment.

COVID and care aesthetics

As has been noted several times during this book, to be writing of care at the time of the Coronavirus pandemic, has made many of the arguments about addressing injustices in access to quality care, or the questions about practices in health, social care and the arts, take on a particular resonance. This has veered from the simple paradox of writing about the art of touch, when touch became a vector of the disease, to exploring the importance of interhuman networked relations when social distance limited them, and the effects of COVID made their fragility even more notable. It is also a global event that has brought the quality and fragility of the care services we all need into sharp relief. The pandemic has shown how care cannot be abstracted from the daily policies of our governments, the strengths and weaknesses of communities and the multiple inequalities that cut through our different contexts. While coming from the UK, there has been a huge amount to be angry about, the focus here will be on moments when positive response might be understood as examples of everyday care aesthetics in action.

In their report on community responses to COVID-19 for the Third Sector Research Centre, based at the University of Birmingham, Angus McCabe, Mandy Wilson, and Rob Macmillan, acknowledge the health and economic impacts of the virus, but then also explain that 'something else seems to be happening' (2021: no page). They show how there have been 'unprecedented levels of informal, often neighbour to neighbour, mutual aid' (Ibid). This takes us right back to the beginning of the book, where the videos showing Italians singing from the balconies in lock down were described. At the time, these films demonstrated something joyfully resistant and how the act of coming out onto the balcony and singing seemed to be an attempt both to find some sense of space for yourself but also reach out to others. While COVID has devastated communities, the image of balcony musicians was, to me, one of the first examples of McCabe and colleague's 'something else happening'.

The 'something else' might have started with balcony singing, but these moments were soon joined by different accounts of local acts of kindness or mutual support. These included baking, as mentioned above, and then shopping and delivering for isolated or shielding neighbours, making signs for windows for creative walks for children, and making home-sewed protective equipment for health professionals. These enter the register of everyday care aesthetics again because rather than a perfunctory effort of providing basic provisions, there were multiple accounts of the special effort people put into the sensory quality of these acts. It was not only cakes and meals that were made with an attention to a certain quality but also the aesthetics of many acts of kindness seemed to reach beyond the demand to meet elementary material needs. One example from early in 2020 was from a friend who set up a network of sewers to create scrubs for health care workers. They were largely machinists from an area in North Manchester where they had traditionally worked in the different clothes factories, and now their skills were gaining recognition and being valued for the contribution to the safety of carers. Again, it was not merely the sewing up of the protective gear and getting it to the staff but also the attention and care with which these garments were made. Their craft of care became a means to reach out and connect to people who, of course, should have had adequate Personal Protective Equipment as part of their employment but who had often been left to fend for themselves by poorly coordinated services. Stepping into a gap with these carefully made scrubs was also an act of artful challenge to the incompetence of our government.

Care aesthetics tracks the way that the execution of a creative act of care is often done with *more than* the basic required as people make an extra effort both for their personal sense of worth but also for how that effort communicates your affection and consideration for the person to whom you are sending the materials. The objects created certainly had an aesthetic quality, so the scrubs, the meals, the cakes, the masks, the care packages, and the shopping bags were frequently prepared with an attention to the sensations they elicited. However, more than in the quality of these objects, care aesthetics is located in the relation that is created between the person, the object and their recipient. This is a restatement of Chapter 1's argument that objects should not be seen as a passive target of aesthetic appreciation, where care for an object might *infer* your care for another, but instead as part of the relation building process as an object *confers* care as it passes from one to another. The interaction that is made possible by these multiple acts becomes the source of the embodied care that is experienced between different people meeting the challenges of a situation. A person-to-person conversation on a doorstep, perhaps an act of kindness while delivering a parcel of goods, is an aesthetic engagement because it is attuned to the sensory needs of both parties, and it has a style, approach, a narrative and regard for the emotional and affective shape of the encounter.

COVID and the arts

Where the end of the last chapter and the beginning of this one explained how an examination of care aesthetics necessarily spills out from the boundaries of the professional to demand an analysis of everyday care aesthetic experiences, COVID gave this tendency an added force. It also demonstrated the spuriousness of the objections to the apparent slippage from aesthetic to social concerns in socially engaged arts practice discussed in Chapter 3, through the speed with which many arts projects embraced the pressing demands of the pandemic. Vafa Ghazavi, a political scientist writing in Deborah Chasman and Joshua Cohen's collection *The Politics of Care: from COVID-19 to Black Lives Matter* (2020), makes an inclusive appeal for social action where 'the moral work is really that of a joint project among many' (Ibid: 49), and certainly arts organisations in the UK at their best have understood themselves as part of a *joint project* and not separate from it. By way of example, Eden Court Highlands in Inverness, Scotland's largest combined arts organisation, turned their 850-seat theatre into a centre for distributing aid, reaching out to their audiences, transforming their services to meet new needs (Gulbenkian, 2021). COVID ensured there was not a debate about the relations between social purpose and aesthetics, but, as explained by François Matarasso in the publication celebrating the Gulbenkian Foundation awards for the cultural sector's response to COVID, the best practices showed organisations 'being part of an interdependent community' where they 'sought ways of putting their human and material resources in the service of all' (Ibid: 6). A particular situation, therefore, demanded that distinctions between *properly* cultural and *properly* caring or social work broke down, and it is not that these organisations became social care agencies, but that the distinction between what was social and what was aesthetic loosened. An organisation that was delivering food parcels *and* art packs was not making two separate offers, but in fact demonstrated a blurring of the line between where the food ended, and the art began.

One noteworthy example from the Gulbenkian publication is called Deveron Projects, from Huntly in Scotland. This arts organisation based in a small town in Aberdeenshire, already had an approach which understood the importance of the everyday, as for them 'art lives in the most ordinary places such as schools, gardens, shops, local landmarks or walking trails' (Ibid: 14). However, their orientation during the early stage of the pandemic was significant for how it linked many of the themes already touched on in this chapter. It is worth quoting the account of their response in full:

> Local shops closed and access to food was immensely compromised, so when questioning what their community needed the most, the conclusion was simple: bread. By mixing art with bread, and seeing bread as art, the Honesty Bakehouse was born. A converted bicycle cart was painted red and carried fresh baked goods for a donation, honestly made with locally sourced ingredients by an artist-turned-baker
>
> *(Ibid: 14–5).*

This was a combined vision that wanted to enrich their community so that it was a place where 'the butcher, the baker and the artist can all live and create together' (Ibid: 15). For the argument for the importance of everyday care aesthetics, it is the insistence on *seeing bread as art* that is most significant, so that there is an aesthetics of routine activities of the everyday, particularly as already discussed above, in the preparation of food. What are not seen in this quotation are the types of interactions and encounters that were made possible through the presence of that converted bicycle cart. The argument here accepts that bread can be art but also seeks to extend this so that it can be the facilitator of caring aesthetic experiences as people share the food, meet over its distribution, and enjoy the sensations of breaking and eating it.

The overall case for everyday care aesthetics suggests care practices operate across multiple parts of our lives, from the professional to the personal, and between the professional and personal. Similarly, the skills bought to aesthetic practices rarely pause as we leave the gallery, studio or theatre, but can imbue our everyday craft practices, such as cooking, mending, or gardening and then more diffusely in how we attend to people, places and objects that exist in our lives. The everyday is, therefore, a particularly fertile site where everyday care and everyday aesthetics merge into each other as, for example, visiting friends, making presents, cooking for neighbours, or reading to children cannot be unpicked to discover where the care ends, and a sensory or aesthetic practice begins. What COVID has done to this argument, however, is to make these tendencies both more notable and more necessary. Eden Court Highlands account for the transformation created during the pandemic by explaining 'for a centre focused on bringing people together, the food parcels offered an alternative, proactive way of connecting with the community' (Ibid: 16). As an echo of Young's social connection model of responsibility, here we have an organisation asserting that this is an obvious extension of their work. As has been suggested throughout this book, this is no flight from a proper artistic role, but an acceptance that bringing people together through the preparation and distribution of food parcels is part of the work of aesthetics: it is an aesthetics of care.

1-1 performers

In previous books, I have written about my own practice, in particular theatre work in prisons, war zones and in other settings. While I was connected to a number of the practical examples in Chapter 3, Care Aesthetics has not been, by and large, an exploration of practices with which I have been intimately involved. Or so I thought. Writing this final chapter on the extension of the case for care aesthetics into everyday life, however, has forced me to consider how it might materialise in my every day. In fact, a number of the examples of cooking, baking and food responses to the pandemic originate with my partner who was involved in cooking for isolating or shielding individuals and establishing a new local bike delivery service during the crisis. I was inspired while writing this by the frequent aesthetically caring examples of practice that emerged in her and her colleagues' efforts.

These issues were highlighted when I was doing an interview with Kirsten Sadeghi-Yekta from Victoria University in Canada for her and Monica Prendergast's book *Applied Theatre: Ethics* (2021) when she asked me *what was my practice now?* I was not working in prisons, not going to war zones, so what creative work was I doing? At first my answer was that I was not involved in practice at the moment, partly explained in my article *To Applied Theatre, with love* (2021), where a move away from professional practice in applied theatre is explained. However, thinking more directly about care aesthetics in the everyday, and a more porous boundary between *where we live our lives* and *where we practice our particular art, craft or caring* has made me reconsider.

During lock down, from its start in the UK in March 2020, up until my writing of the first draft of this chapter in May 2021, I volunteered for a Greater Manchester charity that provides support for struggling families. I acted as mentor for children with different designated special educational needs. At time of writing, I was working with two primary aged children taking them out when rules allowed, giving their parents a break and exploring local parks and their different interests in as an adventurous way as we could under COVID-related restrictions. I was researching care aesthetics during the day and then running around parks, counting squirrels, making dens and defending mounds of dirt from marauding aliens during afternoons and evenings. After Kirsten's question, I had a light bulb moment and realised that this voluntary work was not my afternoon or night off: *this was the thing*. This in turn led to a number of reflections. It made me reconsider the one-to-one performances of Adrian Howells' and the virtuosity of his care aesthetics. It reminded me that we should not dismiss the quality of the one-to-one care of pedicurists, but instead acknowledge the care aesthetics that is made possible in their work, however constrained or undervalued. It then made me realise that one-to-one has been a dominant relational experience for many during COVID as we have been locked in or locked down with a few interpersonal connections. Drawing on these thoughts, I wondered what would happen if we reimagined more of our daily activities, and for me my volunteering, as one-to-one creative care practices.

Work in the socially engaged arts has often been hidden away, in prison classrooms, hospital wards, care homes, refugee camps and so forth. A socially engaged arts version of one-to-one work is similarly hidden. My proposition in this final section of the book is that everyone has been doing 'one-to-one performance' during the Coronavirus pandemic with an aesthetic of care differentially distinguished depending how stressed, over worked or overwhelmed we have been. This includes childcare, parent care, partner care, and student care, whether live or on Zoom. We have not traditionally counted these as one-to-one performance practices but perhaps we do need to claim that they have a sensory, crafted quality. They might just have a certain artistry, or more precisely in the terms used here, they could be considered for their aesthetics. These practices might be hard work, a struggle, or a bit hit and miss, but often they have shot through them a care aesthetics that we should acknowledge and then perhaps seek to nurture.

I cannot claim my one-to-one voluntary work with my young mentees has been hugely skilled. I would argue, however, that it has an aesthetics: a shape and feel, an attempt at a heightened experience and a joint endeavour to create a careful set of sensory, safe activities. While taking place in the urban parks of Manchester, it has been realised as a high energy promenade through imaginary forests and hidden castles. It has included defending park bench ramparts from invisible Minecraft mobs and naming the park's squirrels after online characters. These activities have required a certain attunement, presence, attention to my co-creator, and let's say flexibility with narrative structure that clearly borrowed from skills learnt in years of drama work, and years of childcare. If this is my art practice, then it clearly blurs the boundary between art with a certain carefulness and care with a certain artfulness. And the purpose of mentioning it here is not to suggest it is in any way remarkable but argue that it might have something in common with experiences familiar to other people's everyday lives: lives that are full of activities that we rarely designate as our practice, let alone formally as theatre or drama. Everyday care aesthetics seeks to welcome these types of activity as part of the vision laid out by Ginsborg, who asserts that there is an important everyday politics where relatively small-scale actions 'can have extraordinary cumulative effects' (2005: 49). It seeks to draw attention to, and to value, the creative care that many, if not all of us are involved in. It recognises the baking, shopping, delivering, sewing, and kitchen table lessons forced by school closures. It acknowledges the efforts taken as we seek to bring a style, a richness, a humour and creative sensibility to how we live with and care for our family, friends, neighbours and loved ones. It does not deny that this can be a struggle, but the craft, artistry, and extraordinary virtuosity of artist carers and carer artists involved in these daily practices are more necessary than ever in these difficult times.

Conclusion

Everyday care aesthetics brings this edition to a close. It is the shortest of the chapters here, and yet probably the one that might be the most expansive. On the surface, it suggests that care aesthetics can be significant in all areas of social life. It is important to offer a brief disclaimer on that ambition before seeking to conclude the book. Care aesthetics in the everyday is saying that the moments of interhuman care or carelessness in the world we inhabit need to be analysed for their aesthetics and then practiced with a focus on their sensory quality. It is a search for new forms of connectedness as a resource to meet the many factors that work against individuals acting to support each other and acting to do so in ways that are relationally just and sensorily rich. Too often appeals to our necessary interdependence or the importance of connectedness fail to note that these relations can be blighted not only for their imbalances of power and hierarchies of control but also in the callous, austere or plain boring way they are executed. A dour care home, with time poor and disengaged staff, deserves critique in the same vein that throwing clothes at refugees from a piled-up lorry, and the delivery of food for an elderly person with no word of greeting, or the mutual aid workshop that sends participants to sleep. So, while I do assert the importance of care aesthetics, my disclaimer is that it is only ever a focus within broader analyses and practices, that value, support and seek to realise more equitable and just relations, caring actions and caring arts practices. It is not 'a practice' in and of itself, but a particular aspect of experience, that is shaped by complex systems of economics, social awareness, layered cultures of interhuman behaviour and relations between humans and their material worlds. Care aesthetics points to the sensorily depleted and cruel or, conversely, notes the rich and sensorily dynamic aspects of interpersonal and wider social relations. It does not claim to be anything more than a part of these dynamic systems of reciprocity and care. It rejects the relegation of aesthetics to an incidental icing on a more-weighty social cake, but in presenting it as an integrated aspect of that whole, it does accept that it is only one part of a highly complicated social-aesthetic life world. Even with this disclaimer, my argument is still that it should not be overlooked.

Future care aesthetics

The demand of care aesthetics applies to socially engaged arts projects, suggesting they pay attention to how care for participants, audiences and makers is realised through practice. It inhabits health and social care contexts, pointing to embodied and sensorily well-crafted relations as vital to the experience of that health and care, and finally, it is part of the shape and feel of the relations that strengthen our everyday lives making them more enduring and pleasurable. In many ways this book has merely sketched the aesthetics of care across these areas of life, and the first point, therefore, about future care aesthetics, is the need for more detailed studies of how it relates to specific areas of practice. This requires greater attention to the details of context and to the voice of carers and cared for: that is the presence of those involved in both the receipt and delivery of care in the accounts of those experiences. We need to know the experiences of care aesthetics more precisely, in its different nuances and micro processes, from the perspective of those whose lives are shaped by its importance. This will require ways for capturing and relaying the complexity of interpersonal relations in formal and non-formal contexts, ensuring that it is those at the centre of these experiences who determine the sensations and meanings associated with that practice. These might be micro studies, such as those in Chapter 4 with the Hair and Care project, or the detailed exploration of arts processes, such as workshops or rehearsals. Care aesthetics needs to be put to work as a framework for exploring the dynamics of very different practices, and as a stimulus for the shaping of them.

The second point for future care aesthetics, is to investigate what a cross cultural understanding of the processes might reveal. The introduction of the book examined the poem *Grace* by Roger Robinson, where he recognises the extraordinary care that the nurse Grace enacted in her attention to children, and he reflected that if his son's life *should flicker*, she should be the one to care for him. Robinson's collection, *A Portable Paradise*, is an extraordinary account of Black British experience, and the poem Grace is a vital reminder of the contribution of nurses from the Caribbean to the UK's National Health Service. In *Grace* he offers a poignant account of a practice that has shaped the very style of care that exists in UK health contexts. What is often unnoticed as 'expected' or 'normal' care within our hospital systems, has grown from traditions brought to it from people of colour and professionals with different histories of migration to the UK (I am also thinking here about the practices of nurses from Ireland). Care aesthetics can only be properly understood through a more detailed appreciation of how different communities practice care drawing on a diversity of traditions and cultures. This is not simplistically saying that the aesthetics of care changes in different national or cultural contexts. Saying there is British care, white care, Asian care, Spanish care, or Caribbean care is reductionist and misses the flow of practices across histories and spaces. However, different communities do draw on different assumptions about how bodies relate in space, how physical touch works between individuals and how the voice is used to console or scold. At times this book has referred to the aesthetics of interpersonal relations in Japan, and by extension, care aesthetics needs to be tested through detailed appreciation of the exercise of 'artful care' and 'careful art' in multiple cultural and geographic contexts. This must be with a strongly anti-essentialist, and thus anti-racist intention, whereby the idea of right and wrong, or superior and inferior practices, is firmly rejected, to explore instead the complexity of the patterns of caring aesthetic practices that exist in the artistic and daily lives of diverse communities. This is coupled with the demand that we are humble enough to recognise that we all draw on and are inspired by practices of aesthetically rich care from beyond our immediate experience. On a personal level, by way of a somewhat clichéd example, as a white British man schooled in the handshake as a conduit of affection for another, we must acknowledge that more fulsome embodied methods of welcoming and departing from friends that are now more commonplace (the hug, the kiss on the cheek) are welcome interventions in the care aesthetics of customary British stiffness. Bowlby and colleagues have recognised that 'expressions of emotion through physical affection' are far more common now in the UK and have to some degree replaced a customary 'stiff upper lip' (2010: 169). Care aesthetics needs cross cultural and cross geographic research to understand and appreciate the different aesthetics of interpersonal and inter-communal modes of care. This might map very particular practices in certain highly defined settings, or broader analyses, such as the one suggested above, that might examine how patterns of labour migration transformed the approaches to care across an institution like the National Health Service in the UK.

My final points for future care aesthetics are linked to time and settings. This focus is hinted at in the examples above taken from responses to the Coronavirus pandemic. Care aesthetics needs to be tested through close analysis of practices at particular times, in certain institutions, or applied to certain issues. So detailed study of care aesthetics and the current pandemic but also care aesthetics and past pandemics, for example, the aesthetics of care in response to HIV/AIDS. This might ask, for example, how an aesthetics of deprivation met an aesthetic of care in local or national responses. It might focus on certain institutional settings, so the aesthetics of care in a particular hospital, school or organisation, is traced in detail to explore how people and processes permit relations of care to be nourishing or degrading. It asks what conventions of behaviour, modes of interaction and communication, and then policies facilitate richly crafted networks of creative support, and which do the opposite. Of course, this might be the overall aesthetics of care at play across an arts organisation, related to both the traditional artistic part of the work, and also the total function of the institution. The work of theatre scholars Sarah Bartley (2020) and Caoimhe McAvinchey (2020) on the women and criminal justice focused company, Clean Break Theatre, are excellent examples of this approach. Similarly, it might be an assessment of the aesthetics of care at play across a complete health and social care institution. Of course, it could be an examination of the care aesthetics in an institution which is neither health nor arts related, for example, an aid organisation, a private company or a university. All studies of this type would aim to understand how they were also *of a time*, so that practices would be seen in an historical context, and one that is changing in relation to shifts in practices in local, national or international contexts. Care aesthetics needs it close analysis tied to actual institutions but also it needs its histories, and acknowledgement that it has and will continue to change across time.

A final word

One of the first stories used in the book was an account of my colleague Antoine Muvunyi asking me *why in England people put their children in wheelbarrows*. Following on from above, this is of course a highly perceptive cross-cultural comment on a certain aesthetic of care. While it was an 'incorrect' use of an English word, it was revealing about adult-to-child relations in many European and Western countries. An international colleague, with his simple linguistic slip, managed to shift perspective for those of us for whom *wheelbarrows* were commonplace. His error demonstrated how a focus on care aesthetics can teach us about micro relations that are important for the quality of our lives and how some of the taken for granted practices we rarely note might act as a block on a healthier society.

Children's pushchairs, strollers or prams have never been the same to me since this moment, and I cannot see one now without thinking, in a pastiche of the Communist Manifesto, *we have nothing to lose but our wheelbarrows*. Of course, care aesthetics is not a manifesto that makes this kind of direct, full-throttled demand. The book hopes to draw attention to the aesthetics of care in personal, professional, artistic, health-related and everyday practices, with an ambition to make them richer, more reciprocal, nuanced in execution and respectfully crafted. This might be a modest contribution to building more just and equal relations between individuals, communities and the environments in which they live. At a minimum the depleted care experienced over the months of the Coronavirus pandemic has heightened a realisation that lives would be enriched if we attend to the shape and feel of the caring relations that need to be developed and sustained between us. If this does sound a bit manifesto-like, then so be it. Let's at least question those wheelbarrows and note when carelessness seems to reign there might just be *a spectre haunting our times* which refuses this ugliness. Care aesthetics suggests we *go carefully, for we have a world to win*.

Bibliography

Amigoni, D. and McMullan, G. eds. (2019) *Creativity in Later Life: Beyond Late Style*. London: Routledge.

APPG (2017) *Creative Health: The Arts for Health and Wellbeing. Inquiry Report of the All-Party Parliamentary Group on Art, Health and Wellbeing*. Barnsley: Culture Health and Wellbeing Alliance.

Askins, K. (2014) A quiet politics of being together: Miriam and rose. *Area*, 46(4), pp. 353–4.

Baim, C. (2017) 'The Drama Spiral: A Decision-Making Model for Safe, Ethical, and Flexible Practice When Incorporating Personal Stories in Applied Theatre and Performance', in O'Grady, A. ed. *Risk, Participation and Performance Practice: Critical Vulnerabilities in a Precarious World*. London: Palgrave, pp. 79–109.

Balfour, M. (2019) 'The Politics of Care: Play, Stillness, and Social Presence', in Eckersall, P. and Grehan, H. eds. *The Routledge Companion to Theatre and Politics*. London: Routledge, pp. 93–7.

Bannon, F. (2018) *Considering Ethics in Dance, Theatre and Performance*. London: Palgrave Macmillan.

Barlow Moor Community Association (2021) Stories of Community Solidarity. https://www.sussex.ac.uk/research/projects/groups-and-covid/community-support-and-mutual-aid/stories-mutual-aid-covid-solidarity. Accessed 9/4/21.

Barnes, M. (2015) 'Beyond the Dyad: Exploring the Multidimensionality of Care', in Barnes, M., Brannelly, T., Ward, L. and Ward, N. eds. *Ethics of Care: Critical Advances in International Perspective*. Bristol: Policy Press, pp. 31–44.

Bartley, S. (2020) *Performing Welfare: Applied Theatre, Unemployment and Economies of Participation*. London: Palgrave.

Barton, B. (2014) Performing the paradox of affect and interpretation: Turbulence in vertical city. *Performance Research*, 19(5), pp. 61–8.

Barton, B. and Hansen, P. (2017) 'Risking Intimacy: Strategies of Vulnerability in Vertical City's *All Good Things* and *Trace*', in O'Grady, A. ed. *Risk, Participation and Performance Practice: Critical Vulnerabilities in a Precarious World*. London: Palgrave, pp. 131–52.

Basting, A. (2020) *Creative Care: A Revolutionary Approach to Dementia and Elder Care*. London: HarperOne.

Berleant, A. (2011) *Sensibility and Sense: The Aesthetic Reconstruction of Social Philosophy.* Exeter: Imprint Academic.

Bishop, C. (2012) *Artificial Hells: Participatory Art and the Politics of Spectatorship.* London and New York: Verso.

Bourdieu, P. (1977) *Outline of a Theory of Practice.* Cambridge: Cambridge University Press.

Bourriaud, N. (2002) *Relational Aesthetics.* Trans. Pleasance, S. and Woods, F. with Copeland, M. Dijon: Les Presses du Réel.

Bowden, P. (2008) *Caring: Gender-Sensitive Ethics.* London: Routledge.

Bowlby, S., McKie, L., Gregory, S., & Macpherson, I. (2010). *Interdependency and Care over the Lifecourse.* London: Routledge.

Breunig, K. (1994) 'The Art of Painting Meets the Art of Nursing', in Chinn, P. and Watson, J. eds. *Art and Aesthetics in Nursing.* New York: National League for Nursing Press, pp. 191–201.

Brodzinski, E. (2010) *Theatre in Health and Care.* London: Palgrave Macmillan.

Brykczynska, G. ed. (1997) *Caring: The Compassion and Wisdom of Nursing.* London: Arnold.

Bunting, M. (2020) *Labours of Love: The Crisis of Care.* London: Granta Publications.

Buse, C. and Twigg, J. (2018) Dressing disrupted: Negotiating care through the materiality of dress in the context of dementia. *Sociology of Health & Illness,* 40(2), pp. 340–52.

Butler, J. (2015) *Notes Toward a Performative Theory of Assembly.* Cambridge, MA: Harvard University Press.

Calouste Gulbenkian Foundation (2021) *Celebration 2020-21 – Think About Things Differently.* London: Calouste Gulbenkian Foundation (UK Branch) and Kings College London.

Carper, B. (1978) Fundamental patterns of knowing in nursing. *Advances in Nursing Science,* 1(1), pp. 13–24.

Carter, R. (2007) *The Japanese Arts and Self-Cultivation.* New York: SUNY Press.

Chatterjee, H. ed. (2008) *Touch in Museums: Policy and Practice in Object Handling.* Oxford: Berg.

Chinn, P. and Kramer, M. (2014) *Knowledge Development in Nursing: Theory and Process.* Amsterdam: Elsevier Health Sciences.

Chinn, P. and Watson, J. eds. (1994) *Art and Aesthetics in Nursing.* New York: National League for Nursing Press.

Cooper, C. (2001) *The Art of Nursing: A Practical Introduction.* Philadelphia: Saunders/ Elsevier.

Classen, C. (2020) *The Book of Touch.* London: Routledge.

Clift, S. and Camic, P. eds. (2016) *Oxford Textbook of Creative Arts, Health, and Wellbeing: International Perspectives on Practice, Policy and Research.* Oxford: Oxford University Press.

Contreras Ibacache, V. (2013) Evidence of art in nursing. *Enfermería Global,* 30, pp. 333–8.

Cox, R. (2002) *The Zen Arts: An Anthropological Study of the Culture of Aesthetic Form in Japan.* London: Routledge.

Crawford, P., Brown, B., Baker, C., Tischler, V. and Abrams, B. eds. (2015) *Health Humanities.* London: Palgrave Macmillan.

Crawford, P., Brown, B. and Charise, A. eds. (2020) *The Routledge Companion to Health Humanities.* London: Routledge.

Coutts, M. (2014) *The Iceberg: A Memoire.* London: Atlantic Books.

De Certeau, M. (1984) *The Practice of Everyday Life.* Trans. Randall, S. Berkley: University of California Press.

Dewey, J. (2005) *Art as Experience.* London: Penguin.

Duff Cloutier, J., Duncan, C. and Hill Bailey, P. (2007) Locating Carper's aesthetic pattern of knowing within contemporary nursing evidence, praxis and theory. *International Journal of Nursing Education Scholarship,* 4(1), pp. 1–11.

Elliot–Graves, L. (2021) Healing touch: Using the arts to increase healthy touch between people with PMLD and their carers. *Journal of Applied Arts and Health*, 12(1), pp. 73–85.

England, H. (1986) *Social Work as Art: Making Sense for Good Practice*. London: Allen and Unwin.

Foucault, M. (1990) *The Care of the Self: The History of Sexuality: Volume 3*. Trans. R. Hurley. London: Penguin.

Fredriksson, L. (1999) Modes of relating in a caring conversation: A research synthesis on presence, touch and listening. *Journal of Advanced Nursing*, 30(5), pp. 1167–76.

Gauntlett, D. (2011) *Making Is Connecting: The Social Meaning of Creativity, from DIY and Knitting to You Tube and Web 2.0*. Cambridge: Polity Press.

Ghazavi, V. (2020) 'Ethics at a Distance', in Chasman, D. and Cohen, J. eds. *The Politics of Care: from Covid-19 to Black Lives Matter*. Cambridge: Boston Review in partnership with Verso, pp. 44–50.

Gibson, J. (2020) *Dementia, Narrative and Performance: Staging Reality, Reimagining Identities*. Cham: Palgrave MacMillan.

Gilligan, C. (2009) *In a Different Voice: Psychological Theory and Women's Development*. Cambridge, MA: Harvard University Press.

Gilroy, P. (2004) *After Empire: Melancholia or Convivial Culture*. London: Routledge.

Ginsborg, P. (2005) *The Politics of Everyday Life: Making Choice, Changing Lives*. New Haven and London: Yale University Press.

Gray, M. and Webb, S. (2008) Social work as art revisited. *International Journal of Social Welfare*, 17(1), pp. 182–93.

Groves, R. (2017) 'On Performance and the Dramaturgy of Caring', in Street, A., Alliot, J. and Pauker, M. eds. *Inter Views in Performance Philosophy: Crossings and Conversations*. London: Palgrave, pp. 309–18.

Gulbenkian (2021) *Celebration 2020-21 – Think About Things Differently*. London: Calouste Gulbenkian Foundation (UK Branch) and Kings College London.

Hamera, J. (2011). *Dancing Communities: Performance, Difference and Connection in the Global City*. Basingstoke: Palgrave MacMillan.

Hamington, M. (2004) *Embodied Care: Jane Addams, Maurice Merleau-Ponty, and Feminist Ethics*. Chicago: University of Illinois Press.

Hamington, M. (2010) The will to care: Performance, expectation, and imagination. *Hypatia*, 25(3), pp. 676–95.

Hamington, M. (2011) Care ethics, john Dewey's "Dramatic rehearsal," and moral education. *Philosophy of Education Yearbook 2010*, pp. 121–8.

Hamington, M. (2012) A performative approach to teaching care ethics: A case study. *Feminist Teacher*, 23(1), pp. 31–49.

Hamington, M. (2014) 'Care as Personal, Political, and Performative', in Olthuis, G., Kohlen, H. and Heier, J. eds. *Moral Boundaries Redrawn: The Significance of Joan Tronto's Argument for Political Theory, Professional Ethics, and Care as Practice*. Leuven: Peeters Publishers, pp. 195–212.

Hamington, M. (2015) 'Performing Care Ethics: Empathy, Acting, and Embodied Learning', in Oxley, J. and Ilea, R. eds. *Experiential Learning in Philosophy*. London: Routledge, pp. 52–64.

Hanlon, P., Carlisle, S., Lyon, A. and Hannah, M. (2012) *The Future Public Health*. London: Open University Press.

Hanlon, P. and Carlisle, S. (2016) 'The Fifth Wave of Public Health and the Contributions of Culture and the Arts', in Clift, S. and Camic, P. eds. *Oxford Textbook of Creative Arts, Health, and Wellbeing: International Perspectives on Practice, Policy and Research*. Oxford: Oxford University Press, pp. 19–25.

Harari, D. (2011) Laotang: Intimate encounters. *TDR: The Journal of Performance Studies*, 55(2), pp. 137–149.

Hardt, M. (1999) Affective labor. *Boundary*, 26(2), pp. 89–100.

Hardt, M. and Negri, A. (2004) *Multitude: War and Democracy in the Age of Empire*. London: Penguin.

Hatton, N. (2019) Slowing down: Performance in care homes and the practice of attunement. *RiDE: The Journal of Applied Theatre and Performance*, 24(1), pp. 96–104.

Heddon, D. and Johnson, D. eds. (2016) *It's All Allowed: The Performances of Adrian Howells*. Bristol: Intellect.

Held, V. (2006) *The Ethics of Care: Personal, Political, and Global*. Oxford: Oxford University Press.

Hendry, J. (1993) *Wrapping Culture: Politeness, Presentation, and Power in Japan and Other Societies*. Oxford: Clarendon Press.

Hirsh, E. and Olson, G. (1995) "Je-luce irigaray": A meeting with luce irigaray. Trans. E. Hirsh and G. Brulotte. *Hypatia*, 10(2), pp. 93–114.

Hochschild, A. (1983) *The Managed Heart: The Commercialization of Human Feeling*. Berkley: University of California Press.

Hochschild, A. (2003) *The Commercialization of Intimate Life: Note from Home and Work*. Berkley: The University of California Press.

Hochschild, A. (2012) 'Making Little Things Big', in Smith, P. ed. *The Emotional Labour of Nursing Revisited: Can Nurses Still Care?* Basingstoke: Palgrave MacMillan, pp. xiv–xv.

Hoffman, A. (2020) 'Love One Another or Die', in Chasman, D. and Cohen, J. eds. *The Politics of Care: from Covid-19 to Black Lives Matter*. Cambridge: Boston Review in partnership with Verso, pp. 51–66.

Houston, S. (2020) 'Caring Beyond Illness: An Examination of Godder's Socially Engaged Art and Participatory Dance for Parkinson's Work', in Stuart Fisher, A. and Thompson, J. eds. *Performing Care: New Perspectives on Socially Engaged Performance*. Manchester: Manchester University Press, pp. 69–84.

Hume, N. ed. (1995) *Japanese Aesthetics and Culture: A Reader*. New York: SUNY Press.

Iball, H. (2016) 'Towards and Ethics of Intimate Audiences', in Heddon, D. and Johnson, D. eds. *It's All Allowed: The Performances of Adrian Howells*. Bristol: Intellect.

Ikegami, E. (2005) *Bonds of Civility: Aesthetic Networks and the Political Origins of Japanese Culture*. Cambridge: Cambridge University Press.

Irigaray, L. (2002) *The Way of Love*. Trans Bostic. H. and Pluháček, S. London: Continuum.

Jackson, S. (2011) *Social Works: Performing Art, Supporting Publics*. London: Routledge.

Keady, J., Campbell, S., Clark, A., Dowlen, R., Elvish, R., Jones, L., Kindell, J., Swarbrick, C. and Williams, S. (2020) Re-thinking and re-positioning 'being in the moment' within a continuum of moments: Introducing a new conceptual framework for dementia studies. *Ageing & Society*, pp. 1–22.

Kester, G. (2004) *Conversation Pieces: Community and Communication in Modern Art*. Berkeley: University of California Press.

Kittay, E. (2015) 'A Theory of Justice as Fair Terms of Social Life Given Our Inevitable Dependency and Our Inextricable Interdependency', in Engster, D. and Hamington, M. eds. *Care Ethics and Political Theory*. Oxford: Oxford University Press.

Kongsuwan, W. (2020) Development of the emergent theory of aesthetic nursing practice. *Health*, 12, pp. 764–80.

Lavender, A. (2016) *Performance in the Twenty-First Century: Theatres of Engagement*. London: Routledge.

Leuthold, S. (1998) *Indigenous Aesthetics: Native Art, Media, and Identity*. Austin: University of Texas Press.

Longford, G. (2001) "Sensitive killers, cruel aesthetes, and pitiless poets": Foucault, Rorty, and the ethics of self-fashioning. *Polity*, 33(4), pp. 569–92.

MALB (2020) *Maggie's Architecture and Landscape Brief*. https://www.maggies.org/about-us/publications/. Accessed 14/10/21.

Machon, J. (2017) *Immersive Theatres: Intimacy and Immediacy in Contemporary Performance*. London: Palgrave.

Manning, E. (2007) *Politics of Touch: Sense, Movement, Sovereignty*. Minneapolis: University of Minnesota Press.

Marra, M. (1999) *Modern Japanese Aesthetics: A Reader*. Honolulu: University of Hawai'i Press.

Matarasso, F. (2021) 'Coping – and Changing – With an Existential Crisis', in Calouste Gulbenkian Foundation (2021) *Celebration 2020-21 – Think About Things Differently*. London: Calouste Gulbenkian Foundation (UK Branch) and Kings College London, p. 6.

McAvinchey, C. (2020) *Applied Theatre: Women and the Criminal Justice System*. London: Bloomsbury.

McAvinchey, C. ed. (2013) *Performance and Community: Commentary and Case Studies*. London: Bloomsbury Publishing.

McCabe, A., Wilson, M. and Macmillan, R. (2021) Community responses to Covid-19: early research findings. Local Trust, UK – https://localtrust.org.uk/news-and-stories/blog/community-responses-to-covid-19-early-research-findings. Accessed 9/4/21.

McCann, K. (1993) An examination of touch between nurses and elderly patients in a continuing care setting in Northern Ireland. *Journal of Advanced Nursing*, 18, pp. 838–46.

McCormick, S. (2017) *Applied Theatre: Creative Ageing*. London: Bloomsbury Publishing.

Merleau-Ponty, M. (2013) *Phenomenology of Perception*. Trans. Landes, D. London: Routledge.

Miles, M. (2011) *Herbert Marcuse: An Aesthetics of Liberation*. London: Pluto Press.

Miner, D. (2017) *Indigenous Aesthetics: Art, Activism, and Autonomy*. London: Bloomsbury.

Moss, H. and O'Neil, D. (2014) The art of medicine: Aesthetic deprivation in clinical settings. *The Lancet*, 383, pp. 1032–3.

Moss, H. (2020) 'Aesthetics of Space', in Crawford, P., Brown, B. and Charise, A. eds. *The Routledge Companion to Health Humanities*. London: Routledge, pp. 430–5.

Murphy, K. (2020) Braiding borders: Performance as care and resistance on the US-Mexico border. *TDR: The Journal of Performance Studies*, 64(4), pp. 72–83.

Myers, E. (2013) *Worldly Ethics: Democratic Politics and Care for the World*. Durham, NC: Duke University Press.

Nanay, B. (2019) *Aesthetics: A Very Short Introduction*. Oxford: Oxford University Press.

Nayeri, D. (2018) 'Accepting Charity is an Ugly Business': my return to the refugee camps, 30 years on. Guardian Newspaper – 15/9/2018.

Noddings, N. (2013) *Caring: A Relational Approach to Ethics and Moral Education*. Berkley: University of California Press.

Nussbaum, M. (2010) 'Foreword', in Young, I. ed. *Responsibility for Justice*. Oxford: Oxford University Press, pp. ix–xxv.

O'Grady, A. ed. (2017) *Risk, Participation and Performance Practice: Critical Vulnerabilities in a Precarious World*. London: Palgrave.

Orozco, L. (2017) 'Theatre in the Age of Uncertainty: Memory, Technology, and Risk in Simon McBurney's *The Encounter* and Robert Lepage's *887*', in O'Grady, A. ed. *Risk, Participation and Performance Practice: Critical Vulnerabilities in a Precarious World*. London: Palgrave, pp. 33–55.

Parsons, G. and Carlson, A. (2008) *Functional Beauty*. Oxford: Oxford University Press.

Paterson, M. (2006) 'Affecting Touch: Towards a 'Felt' Phenomenology of Therapeutic Touch', in Bondi, L. and Davidson, J. eds. *Emotional Geographies*. London: Routledge.

Philips, J. (2007) *Care*. Cambridge: Polity Press.

Pink, S. (2012) *Situating Everyday Life: Practices and Places*. London: SAGE Publications.

Pink, S., Morgan, J. and Dainty, A. (2014) The safe hand: Gels, water, gloves and the materiality of tactile knowing. *Journal of Material Culture*, 19(4), pp. 425–42.

Puig de la Bellacasa, M. (2017) *Matters of Care: Speculative Ethics in More than Human Worlds*. Minnesota: University of Minnesota Press.

Rancière, J. (2004) *The Politics of Aesthetics*. Trans G. Rockhill. London: Continuum.

Robinson, F. (1999) *Globalizing Care: Ethics, Feminist Theory, and International Relations*. Boulder: Westview Press.

Robinson, F. (2011) *The Ethics of Care: A Feminist Approach to Human Security*. Philadelphia: Temple University Press.

Robinson, R. (2019) *A Portable Paradise*. Leeds: Peepal Tree Press.

Rovithis, M. (2002) Nursing as an art. *ICUs and Nursing Web Journal*, 9, pp. 1–14.

Sadeghi-Yekta, K. and Prendergast, M. (2022) *Applied Theatre: Ethics*. London: Bloomsbury.

Saito, Y. (2008) *Everyday Aesthetics*. Oxford: Oxford University Press.

Saito, Y. (2017) *Aesthetics of the Familiar: Everyday Life and World-Making*. Oxford: Oxford University Press.

Sedgwick, E. K. (2003) *Touching Feeling: Affect, Pedagogy, Performativity*. Durham: Duke University Press.

Sevenhuijsen, S. (2003) *Citizenship and the Ethics of Care: Feminist Considerations on Justice, Morality and Politics*. London: Routledge.

Shaughnessy, N. (2012) *Applying Performance: Live Art, Socially Engaged Theatre and Affective Practice*. London: Palgrave.

Schusterman, R. (2000) *Performing Live: Aesthetic Alternatives for the Ends of Art*. New York: Cornell University Press.

Shusterman, R. (2012) *Thinking through the Body*. Cambridge: Cambridge University Press.

Siles-González, J. and Solano-Ruiz, C. (2016) Sublimity and beauty: A view from nursing aesthetics. *Nursing Ethics*, 23(2), pp. 154–66.

Smith, P. (2012) *The Emotional Labour of Nursing Revisited: Can Nurses Still Care?* Basingstoke: Palgrave MacMillan.

Swarbrick, C., Keady, J. and Sampson, E. (2017) Notes from the hospital bedside: Reflections on researcher roles and responsibilities at the end of life in dementia. *Quality in Ageing and Older Adults*, 18(3), pp. 201–11.

Stuart Fisher, A. and Thompson, J. eds. (2020) *Performing Care: New Perspectives on Socially Engaged Performance*. Manchester: Manchester University Press.

Tahhan, D. (2014) *The Japanese Family: Touch, Intimacy, and Feeling*. London: Routledge.

Tanner, L. (2017) *Embracing Touch in Dementia Care: A Person-Centred Approach to Touch and Relationships*. London: Jessica Kingsley Publishers.

The Care Collective (2020) *The Care Manifesto: The Politics of Interdependence*. London: Verso.

Thompson, J. (2009) *Performance Affects: Applied Theatre and the End of Effect*. London: Palgrave.

Thompson, J. (2014) *Humanitarian Performance: from Disaster Tragedies to Spectacles of War*. Chicago: Seagull/University of Chicago Press.

Thompson, J. (2015) Towards an aesthetics of care. *RiDE: The Journal of Applied Theatre and Performance*, 20(4), pp. 1–12.

Thompson, J. (2017) No more bystanders: 'Grandchildren of Hiroshima' and the 70th anniversary of the atomic bomb. *TDR: The Journal of Performance Studies*, 61(2), pp. 87–104.

Thompson, J. (2020) 'Performing the "aesthetics of Care"', in Stuart Fisher, A. and Thompson, J. eds. *Performing Care: New Perspectives on Socially Engaged Performance*. Manchester: Manchester University Press, pp. 215–29.

Thompson, J. (2021) *To applied theatre, with love. TDR: The Journal of Performance Studies.* 65(1), pp. 167–79.

Thompson, N. ed. (2012) *Living as Form: Socially Engaged Art 1991-2011.* Cambridge, MA: MIT Press.

Tronto, J. (1993) *Moral Boundaries: A Political Argument for an Ethic of Care.* London: Routledge.

Tronto, J. (2013) *Caring Democracy: Markets, Equality, and Justice.* New York: New York University Press.

Twigg, J. (2000) Carework as a form of bodywork. *Ageing and Society,* 20, pp. 389–411.

Twigg, J. (2002) *Bathing - the Body and Community Care.* London: Routledge.

Twigg, J., Wolkowitz, C., Cohen, R. and Nettleton, S. eds. (2011) *Body Work in Health and Social Care: Critical Themes, New Agendas.* London: Wiley.

Twigg, J. and Martin, W. eds. (2015) *Routledge Handbook of Cultural Gerontology.* London: Routledge.

Wainwright, P. (2000) Towards an aesthetics of nursing. *Journal of Advanced Nursing,* 32(3), pp. 750–6.

Wake, C. (2017) The ambivalent politics of one-to-one performance. *Performance Paradigm: a Journal of Performance and Contemporary Culture,* 17, pp. 163–173.

Ward, R., Campbell, S. and Keady, J. (2014) 'Once I had money in my pocket, I was every colour under the sun': Using 'appearance biographies' to explore the meanings of appearance for people with dementia. *Journal of Aging Studies,* 30, pp. 64–72.

Ward, R., Campbell, S. and Keady, J. (2016a) Assembling the salon: Learning from alternative forms of body work in dementia care. *Sociology of Health & Illness,* 38(8), pp. 1287–302.

Ward, R., Campbell, S. and Keady, J. (2016b) 'Gonna make yer gorgeous': Everyday transformation, resistance and belonging in the care-based hair salon. *Dementia,* 15(3), pp. 395–413.

Welton, M. (2013) 'Rosemary Lee: Interview and Introduction', in McAvinchey, C. ed. (2013) *Performance and Community: Commentary and Case Studies.* London: Bloomsbury Publishing, Loc, pp. 2343–528.

Western, R. (2017) 'At the Risk of Being Sincere: Participation and Delegation in South African Contemporary Live Art', in O'Grady, A. ed. *Risk, Participation and Performance Practice: Critical Vulnerabilities in a Precarious World.* London: Palgrave, pp. 179–204.

Young, M. (2010) *Responsibility for Justice.* Oxford: Oxford University Press.

Zontou, Z. (2017) '*Upon Awakening:* Addiction, Performance, and Aesthetics of Authenticity', in O'Grady, A. ed. *Risk, Participation and Performance Practice: Critical Vulnerabilities in a Precarious World.* London: Palgrave, pp. 205–31.

INDEX

For Product Safety Concerns and Information please contact our EU
representative GPSR@taylorandfrancis.com Taylor & Francis Verlag GmbH,
Kaufingerstraße 24, 80331 München, Germany

Printed and bound by CPI Group (UK) Ltd, Croydon, CR0 4YY

08/06/2025

01897006-0019